When You're Sick

and Don't Know Why

Coping with Your Undiagnosed Illness

Linda Hanner, John J. Witek, M.D.
with Robert B. Clift, Ph.D.

When Your Sick and Don't Know Why © 1991
by Linda Hanner, John J. Witek, with Robert B. Clift

Library of Congress Cataloging-in-Publication Data

Hanner, Linda.
    When you're sick and don't know why; coping with your undiagnosed illness/Linda Hanner, John J. Witek,
    with Robert B. Clift.
        p.   cm.
    Includes bibliographical references and index.
    ISBN 0-937721-83-2: $9.95
    1. Chronic diseases. 2. Sick—Psychology.
    3. Adjustment (Psychology)
    I. Witek, John J. II. Clift, Robert B. III. Title.
RC108.H36   1991
155.9'16—dc20   91-13852   CIP

Edited by: Donna Hoel
Cover Design: Nancy Bolmgren
Text Design/Production Manager: Wenda Johnson
Printed in the United States of America

10 9 8 7 6 5 4 3 2 1

Published by:

DCI Publishing
P.O. Box 47945
Minneapolis, MN 55447-9727

DEDICATION

To my husband, Kim, and my children, Jerimiah, Jason, Jennifer, and Jonathan, for their love and patience.

FOREWORD

To be ill is a trial under any circumstances, but to be ill and not know the cause is a particularly great affliction. The burden imposed by such a situation is not merely being without access to a cure. There's the added fear of the unknown, isolation from not knowing other people who have gone through the same thing and, worst, self-blame, aided by the medical profession's failure to understand what you're experiencing.

Mysterious illness is likewise disquieting to doctors. Finding a diagnosis brings mutual satisfaction for doctor and patient— best, of course, if there is a cure as well. All too often the answer "I don't know" is unacceptable to both doctor and patient; there's the feeling that the doctor *ought* to know.

A patient who for unknown reasons continues to suffer can trigger in the physician a sense of failure— or at the very least, an uncomfortable awareness of the limitations of his or her knowledge and power. At worst, the doctor might blame the patient in some way or discount what the patient has to say. A situation of mutual animosity can develop, in which the patient becomes increasingly desperate and angry and the physician increasingly defensive and unheeding.

Linda Hanner's book is a step toward breaking this deadlock. She uses her own experience with undiagnosed Lyme disease to affirm that the doctor and patient's ability to work together in the face of a mutual unknown enemy is in itself of tremendous value. She outlines strategies for getting the most help possible from the medical profession and for minimizing the trauma that results from misunderstanding. Dr. Witek explains the limitations inherent in medical practice and helps patients form realistic expectations of their doctors and perhaps reduce animosity when uncertainty persists.

While she never downplays the difficulties, Linda Hanner comes through loud and clear with a message of hope, one she found in her personal experience and again in talking with others. Furthermore, through her writing, she has found a way to help. She gives many practical suggestions to help patients learn to negotiate their way through the formidable and complicated health-care system, as well as through alternative health care. She shares her own and others' experience as a way to help people cope— with their own emotions and, indeed, with living with an undiagnosed illness. And she implicitly offers what most people need in the absence of a diagnosis and cure: respect and validation for what they are going through.

Reading about Ms. Hanner's experience, as well as those of other people she quotes, should help sufferers to feel less isolated. Others, too, have trod the lonely path of undiagnosed illness, have lived for months or years with uncertainty, have grieved the changes in their functional capacities and in their relationships. Others, too, have felt, at times, that when needed most, doctors, friends, and family members have seemed to be enemies: blaming, disbelieving, uncomprehending.

This is a much-needed book. Different parts of it will likely strike a particular resonance with different people. There should be something in it for almost anyone faced with undiagnosed illness, whether it's a story or vignette you can relate to, a practical tip leading to a diagnosis, a more effective management of pain, or the articulation of a hope or belief to hold to and live by, even in the midst of illness and uncertainty.

Jenifer A. Nields, M.D.
Yale University, New Haven, Connecticut

ACKNOWLEDGEMENTS

T he willingness of so many people to share their stories and the generous contributions of several medical professionals helped make this book possible. I wish to especially acknowledge and thank the following people:

Dr. John Witek for believing in the value of this project and agreeing to co-author it.

Dr. Robert Clift, who reinforced my belief in the need for this book, spent many hours reviewing the manuscript, and offered valuable personal insight.

Carol Frick, my friend and educator, who has encouraged me in this and all my writing endeavors and has inspired confidence in me.

Dr. Jenifer Nields and Dr. Brian Fallon for carefully reading the manuscript and giving expert advice and important personal perspectives.

Brad and Lynn Schmidt for sharing their story and the many others who contributed excerpts and insights from their experiences with undiagnosed medical problems.

Linda Hanner

Contents

Introduction

I became aware of the tremendous need for this book during my own six-year bout with an undiagnosed illness and as a result of the hundreds of calls and letters I have received since the publication of my first book, *Lyme Disease: My Search for a Diagnosis.** I continue to hear from victims of a wide array of illnesses ranging from cancer to rheumatoid arthritis, thanking me for sharing my experience. Many of them say, "You've written my story."

Those who now have answers express gratitude that someone has put into words what they felt before the diagnosis. Those who are still searching say that knowing someone else can identify with their pain has helped lighten their load and given them a sense of hope.

My illness came as an unwelcome and terrifying intruder in the midst of a fast-paced but relatively predictable lifestyle. During the ensuing six years of bizarre and fluctuating symptoms I struggled to hang onto my faith and my sanity. The symptoms disrupted my life and the lives of my husband and children.

*The original title of this book, published in 1989, was **Of Power & Love & Sound Mind: Six Years with Undiagnosed Lyme Disease.**

For years I spent a great deal of time poring over medical books and reading every article about specific diseases I could lay my hands on, hoping to find clues, connections, or some kind of explanation for my problems. I never considered reading a self-help book for victims of chronic illness. My focus was on finding an answer, not on learning to live with my condition. Even though I felt sick and was unable to function normally most of the time, I was always uncertain whether my illness was real or a figment of my imagination.

When doctors suggested my symptoms were psychological, I knew in my heart they were wrong, yet the same questions rolled over and over in my mind: Why can't anyone come up with an answer? What's wrong with me? I struggled with guilt. I became frustrated and angry with the medical profession. I felt there was no one else who could understand my predicament. I was, at times, even jealous of others who returned from a doctor's appointment with a diagnosis.

Finally, after four years of struggling, I came to a point of acceptance. I realized I may never have a name for my illness, but that didn't matter so much anymore. Ironically, it was during a prescription drug-induced psychotic episode in which every ounce of my credibility had been stripped away that I started to really believe in myself. I became convinced of my own mental stability.

My faith in God and myself became most important to me. I knew I didn't want or need to be sick—I just was. And I started dealing with it one day at a time. I found a place of peace and comfort in the midst of my uncertainty. I stopped feeling like a victim. I realized I couldn't control what was happening to my body, nor could I control the opinions of others; I could only be myself. I gained self-confidence and became more assertive. I allowed myself to become angry and then moved beyond the anger to find a sense of purpose. I learned to focus on other people and events, rather than on my own body.

My circumstances hadn't changed, but I found it easier to cope. Even as my physical symptoms worsened, I felt emotionally and spiritually well. When I finally received my diagnosis and was successfully treated for Lyme disease, it was an added blessing.

During my bout with Lyme disease I learned a great deal about myself, about human relationships, about the power of God, about medical science, and about difficult-to-diagnose illnesses.

Dr. John Witek, a dedicated and caring neurologist, became involved in my case during the last two years of my illness and was immensely helpful to me. Through the relationship we developed I discovered it is possible for doctors and patients to work together as a team. Dr. Witek stood out among the rest, not because of greater knowledge but because he respected my feelings, was honest about the limitations of medical science, consistently allowed my input in decision making, and offered empathy and encouragement. When I realized the value of a physician's input in writing this book, I was honored and pleased that Dr. Witek felt it a worthy task and agreed to help.

A third person involved in this project was Dr. Robert Clift, a clinical psychologist who frequently counsels patients with undiagnosed physical problems and who also believed strongly in the value of this endeavor.

Although most of this book is written from my point of view, I have incorporated the knowledge and suggestions of these two professionals. Chapter 2 was written entirely by Dr. Witek. Through our combined efforts—my personal experience and the knowledge and skills of both professionals—we have explored the various aspects of undiagnosed illness.

In *When You're Sick and Don't Know Why* it is our intention to address the deep psychological pain of the many sufferers of undiagnosed illness and to inject insight into the doctor-patient relationship by exploring the expectations and frustrations of individuals on both sides of the issue.

Our goals for this book are to offer comfort, hope, and practical advice to those of you who are suffering from undiagnosed illness. We hope it will help you to sort out the physical and psychological components of your illness and to effectively communicate your needs to your doctor, family, and friends. Most important, we hope it will help you believe in yourself and find the strength to cope with your condition and your uncertainty. We have included information that will help you understand why it often takes time to diagnose symptoms and why sometimes a diagnosis is not possible.

Although the pain and frustration I experienced during my own struggle with undiagnosed illness often seem remote to me now, each time I receive a call or letter from one of you my memories are refreshed. Your anguish comes through loud and clear, as well as your gratitude that someone is willing to listen.

I would never have chosen to go through what I did, but I can honestly say I am not sorry for anything that happened. I learned so much and believe I am much stronger in many ways because of it. I became acutely aware of the limitations of medical science, and at the same time sincerely impressed with how much it has to offer. I pray that this book will be helpful and encouraging to those who are still struggling.

Linda Hanner

CHAPTER 1

The Hardest Part Is Not Knowing

The happiest day of my life was the day the doctors at the Mayo Clinic told me I had MS. The five years before that—the years I didn't know what was wrong—were the worst years of my life. I was sick, but no one believed me. The doctors shoved antidepressants and tranquilizers at me. Even my mother accused me of being a kitchen drunk.

—Lil

O nly those who have lived for months or years with the anguish of an undiagnosed illness can fully understand the relief and joy of finally getting a diagnosis— even when the prognosis isn't good.

Chronic illnesses are painful, unpredictable, and depressing. They stress family relationships, undermine careers, and spoil activities you enjoyed in the past. However, once you have a diagnosis you also have the possibility of treatment and recovery, or at least some structure for reordering your life.

The uniquely cruel aspect of undiagnosed illness is that, even though the pain and devastation are very real, there's the underlying suspicion of doctors, family, well-meaning friends, and ultimately even you that the cause is psychological. Blaming the victim is often the next step when medical training and technology prove inadequate. Until the diagnosis there are only uncertainties, self-doubt, and continuous questions.

I recall waking up every day in pain. I would try to convince myself nothing was wrong and to force my body to do what it refused to do. I kept asking myself, "Am I sick or crazy? Am I bringing this on myself? If I am healthy, why do I hurt so bad, and why can't I function as I did before."

At any given moment, millions of people are in the predicament of being sick without knowing why. In fact, when people go through medical exams, more than half the time they don't receive clear-cut explanations for their symptoms.[1]

Of the hundreds of people with diagnosed chronic illnesses who I interviewed while writing this book, the vast majority said it took a long time— often months or years— for their illnesses to be diagnosed. They also said the period of time between the first appearance of symptoms and an accurate diagnosis was very difficult.

If you are a victim of undiagnosed illness, chances are you can understand the fear, self-doubt, anger, and frustration that so often accompany it. Although you may feel alone and isolated, you can be assured there are many others out there like you.

You and your family may feel as though you're on an emotional roller coaster. There may be times when your symptoms temporarily subside and you're almost convinced they were a figment of your imagination— or at least not as bad as you thought. But when they return with a vengeance a short time later, you know you're not making them up.

Your symptoms might include pain, weakness, fatigue, and other problems that are not readily apparent to people around you. Your doctor might detect few or no objective signs of illness and can only go by what you say.

The doctor might attribute your symptoms to some sort of virus, but if those symptoms have persisted for several months with no explanation, he or she might suggest stress or depression as a cause. The doctor might advise you to forget about your symptoms and exercise or socialize more. But you simply can't take your mind off them. You feel your doctor has abandoned you just when you need him or her the most.

If you have tended to be a workaholic in the past, your friends and family might be concerned that overwork caused your illness. They tell you if you don't rest more, then it's your own fault you aren't getting better. You hear remarks such as, "You mean they still haven't figured out what's wrong with you?" Others begin to doubt you.

In defense, you clam up and refuse to talk about your condition at all. Or you become obsessive about your symptoms and talk about them too much, feeling that if only you could convince people that something is really physically wrong with you, someone would be able to help.

Even if you have been able to drag yourself to work every day, you worry about the future because you just don't know how much longer you will be able to keep going. You have tried to talk your symptoms away, tried to ignore them, and tried to force yourself to do things you couldn't do. Meanwhile, you feel as though you are in a snowballing cycle of fear, anxiety, and self-doubt. Although you once saw yourself as a reasonably confident, capable person, you now feel helpless and confused.

When a medical evaluation fails to reveal an organic explanation for your symptoms, it's disconcerting for both you and your health-care providers. In these situations it is not uncommon for doctors to turn to psychological explanations. Although emotional factors do play a role in any illness, many patients and doctors agree that the modern medical profession tends at times to go overboard in assuming the entire cause of most undiagnosed illnesses is psychological.

I have talked with many lay people who have become intimidated and distrustful of the medical profession. Examples of situations where patients were misunderstood by doctors continued to fall in my lap before and throughout the writing of this book. It seems as if everyone has a doctor story to tell, either about themselves or a friend or family member.

The scenarios include victims of significant physical problems that didn't show up on tests for a long time, had no tests available, or didn't follow patterns typical of the disease causing them. In other instances the doctors didn't make a diagnosis simply because they refused to take the patients' complaints seriously.

In difficult-to-diagnose situations it's especially important for doctors and patients to work together as a team. Doctors need to be open-minded and give patients more credit for knowing when something is wrong with their own bodies. Patients need to understand it's not always possible for doctors to provide the answers they would like to have. In spite of years of medical training, doctors aren't capable of knowing everything that's going on inside a patient's body. They can't feel what the patient is feeling. Besides the more obvious illnesses that are sometimes overlooked, many illnesses are notorious for being difficult to diagnose, and there are many unknowns in medical science.

Although "the doctor knows best" and "follow the doctor's orders" have become common cliches, doctors don't always know best, and the verdicts they come up with aren't always accurate. Very often when two doctors are consulted for the same problem, they come up with conflicting diagnoses. Obviously they can't both be right. Most doctors' decisions are based on educated guesses, which are subject to error.

Society assigns doctors the roles of judge and jury when it comes to illness. This has resulted in most of us erroneously believing that when we have symptoms causing concern or disrupting our lifestyle, the doctor will find the cause and offer a remedy. We then become disconcerted and feel let down when that doesn't happen.

> *I was angry, scared, and hurt. I knew I was really sick, but until I proved it, I was afraid no one would help me. I felt isolated and confused. I worried that my family and friends would reject me. I knew there had to be an answer somewhere. There just had to! But I didn't know where to turn.*
> *—Irene (arthritis victim)*

Somehow, whether or not a diagnosis is reached, each patient must come to terms with his or her illness and find ways to cope. In Chapter 2 we will explain some of the many reasons illnesses go undiagnosed. In the remaining chapters we will offer advice on increasing your chances of being diagnosed, and we'll explore ways to help you and your family start managing and coping while you're in limbo. When you and your family accept and understand your situation, it will be less painful and much more hopeful.

CHAPTER 2

Why Doctors Can't Diagnose Your Illness

This chapter, written by John J. Witek, M.D., a neurologist, provides insights into the physician's perspective.

M edical diagnosis— seems it should be straightforward and simple. You have some symptoms, so you go to the doctor and are examined. Possibly some tests are done, then you're given the diagnosis and treatment plan. Yet that isn't always the case.

Most of us have been conditioned to expect dramatic results when it comes to health care. On TV, even obscure diseases are diagnosed and treated in 60 minutes— minus commercials! Wouldn't it be nice if that were true in real life?

In many cases, the diagnostic process involves a series of complex steps. Lots of information has to be obtained, sorted, and organized before any conclusions can be drawn. Difficulties arise because of problems with information collection and analysis; limitations of physicians, laboratories, or diagnostic procedures; and lack of medical knowledge.

New disease processes continue to be identified, with AIDS and Lyme disease being two of the most widely publicized in recent years. Research uncovers new information that makes it necessary to modify or radically change old ideas and concepts. Medical science today is neither complete nor perfect— nor will it be anytime in the foreseeable future.This chapter will explain some of the potential pitfalls in medical diagnosis and why diagnostic tests don't always give answers— and can in fact be misleading.

To start, some definitions might be helpful. A *symptom* is something experienced or felt by the patient; it's therefore subjective. A *sign* is an objective manifestation or physical finding the physician detects during the examination. Symptoms can sometimes also be associated with objective signs and are then verifiable by the physician.

Diagnosis is a term derived from Greek words meaning to distinguish or discern. In the past, the word meant symptoms and signs by which a disease could be recognized. Today it means the process of identifying a disease by investigation of its symptoms, signs, and other manifestations. What's actually happening in the doctor's office is the attempt to decide if the patient's problem is due to disease A, disease B, disease C, or something else. This is *differential diagnosis*, and we'll talk more about that later.[1]

Medical Consultation: The Process and Potential Pitfalls

What really occurs when a patient consults a physician? It begins with a person telling the story of a symptom or symptoms that have been occurring for a period of time. This story may be highly refined and detailed, or it may be more of a rough draft, depending on how many times it's been told and how inquisitive listeners have been. Ideally, patients should be given adequate time to relate their stories (or their child's or relative's story) in their own words. Unfortunately, economic forces, administrative pressures, and other factors have cut into the amount of time available for each patient. Studies have shown that physicians allow only nine minutes, on average, for history taking.[2] Also, patients often report they are interrupted within 30 seconds of starting to talk. If a medical problem is complex or elusive, lack of time can be a problem.

In addition to time, a number of other factors conspire against the task of transferring information from patient to physician. Describing symptoms can be very difficult. It may seem cut and dried to say you've been having headaches, pain, numbness, weakness, or dizziness, but these words have different meanings for each of us. The doctor needs to understand each symptom as thoroughly as possible. And each symptom can trigger a number of additional questions.

The first time you see the doctor, he or she may ask: When did this symptom begin? Is it constant or variable? How often is it occurring? Is the frequency changing? Are there any other factors that seem to play a role, such as certain activities or positions, stress, fatigue, meals or missed meals, medications (prescription or over-the-counter), etc? You answer as carefully as you can. But then you probably go home and reconsider the symptoms in light of what was asked. You might even begin keeping a diary so you can provide more specific details next time. (That's a good idea, by the way.)

If you're at a point where you've seen a number of doctors and polished your story through repetition, you may also be at a disadvantage. Perhaps you've sensed some information was unimportant to the last four or five physicians you talked with, and now you automatically leave that out. Yet this subjective elimination of information may not be in your best interest. The very piece of information one doctor takes lightly may strike another physician as crucial.

The History

The initial history-taking is critical. Information obtained will color everything that follows, including the physical exam, lab and other tests, and follow-up visits. Without an accurate and reasonably thorough information base, the likelihood of failure or error in diagnosis obviously rises.

In most cases, the majority of history-taking occurs at the first visit. Any information not acquired then may be unavailable to the physician for some time. Missing facts may surface later, but in some cases failure to acquire all available information at the first contact could lengthen the diagnostic process. As a patient, you need to be prepared to share as much information as you possibly can.

While the patient is providing information, a number of things are probably happening inside the physician's head. Nonverbal clues are important, and much can be gleaned from observation. The patient's appearance, demeanor, interactions, and whether or not their presentation in the office is consistent with the type and severity of the symptoms reported can be crucial in understanding both the patient and the problem. The style and coherence of the story can give some insights into the patient.

The physician is also going to have to form an opinion as to the reliability of the information being provided by the patient. Some estimation of the patient's mental competence is needed. Each person observes and describes symptoms differently. Also, state of mind affects our ability to convey information clearly. It's not unusual for a patient to be anxious during an office visit. And anxiety can be amplified when the patient needs to discuss long-standing and disruptive symptoms. It can be very difficult to convey a medical history satisfactorily and even more difficult to provide a concise and well thought-out response to questions.

The Physical

Physical examination usually follows the interview. Depending on the symptoms and the type of physician consulted, this could be general or selective, such as an eye, ear, heart, or nervous system exam. It's possible to examine for a tremendous number of physical findings— but not very practical. In most cases, the physician tailors the exam for that person's particular symptoms, possibly combined with some personal observations. Certain findings or the lack of findings (an absent sign can be important!) may change the course of the exam.

Now the physician's judgement becomes paramount. The ability to adapt the physical examination, based on history and evolving information, is a skill honed over years of medical practice. It allows physicians to judge which areas will be screened or omitted and which will be pursued in depth.

Obtaining critical information from an examination can be difficult. Physical findings or signs can be fleeting or intermittent (as can the subjective symptoms reported by the patient) and may not be apparent at the time of consultation. Potentially useful information can easily be missed if part of an examination is omitted because the doctor judged it unnecessary based on available information.

Deciding whether a finding is normal or abnormal can be quite challenging, since the range of normal is, at times, impressive. In my neurology practice, for example, I must often determine whether reflexes are normal or abnormal. A well-muscled individual will tend to have relatively inactive or quiet reflexes. In contrast, someone who is anxious may appear to have hyperactive reflexes because of increased nervous system activity associated with anxiety. Thus a physician must cautiously interpret findings and also look for extenuating factors, such as those mentioned. Over time, I've learned that an isolated but definite physical finding, though it can't be ignored, may not be important. On the other hand, a series of subtle signs that appear to fall within the "broad range of normal" can sometimes be tied together and lead toward a definitive diagnosis.

A physical finding may not be related to the problem at hand. Maybe it's part of a previous illness or condition— presumably identified during the history-taking. Also, in some cases, more than one medical problem may be present, and this can confound the diagnostic process. And finally, sometimes it's just not possible to ascribe symptoms to a specific medical problem.

Sorting It Out

Once the physical exam is completed, the physician can attempt to formally analyze the combined history and physical findings. Of course, this process isn't suddenly switched on; it's continuous, beginning with the first contact with the patient. I can still clearly remember listening to case discussions during my neurology training. The discussions often began, "This is a 36-year-old man . . ." At that point, the head of the neurology department would say, "Stop! What possible problems are common in a man in his 30s?" The discussion would move on from there, and each bit of information would raise similar questions.

My point, of course, is that every bit of information can be helpful and must be carefully considered. Even more importantly, if any information is going to be discarded, this must be done cautiously and with some capability to recall it if necessary. The ongoing analysis permits us to reconsider earlier impressions and begin to build a list of possible diagnoses.

The first step in the analysis is to look at each bit of information and rate its possible significance. The doctor decides which symptoms are pertinent and which are not; some symptoms may be merely coincidental. The medical history may suggest that previous, possibly unrelated, medical problems explain some of the findings. Or perhaps the current medical problem is related to an earlier problem, which may or may not have been recognized in the past. If that prior problem was diagnosed, can we accept that diagnosis as accurate?

The next step is to review facts thought to be most important. Data might be organized around a central fact or two— possibly a major symptom or obviously important physical finding. The real skill is to now look at all the other facts and try to discern if any or all of them can be grouped as part of a particular disorder or syndrome. Even when a certain sign or symptom is a specific marker for one disease and only one disease, it's necessary to determine if that diagnosis can satisfactorily explain all the other facts.

In most cases, the facts won't fit neatly under a single disease process. It may then be necessary to consider a list of possible diagnoses or a "differential diagnosis." Probability factors can be assigned to each of the possibilities, based on the physician's knowledge of the possible disorders and their frequencies of occurrence. Factors such as age, sex, race, and country of origin also may be important. When considering the probabilities, many physicians have been taught the clinical adage, "When one hears hoofbeats, think of horses and not zebras." That's at least true here in the U.S. In other words, common things occur frequently, uncommon things don't.

Next the physician begins to narrow the list down. This often is termed "ruling in" or "ruling out" a particular diagnosis. More lab tests or other procedures may be needed, or the physician might decide more time is needed to watch the progress of the symptoms.

I hope I've explained how incredibly complex the diagnostic process can be. Yet I don't want to create the impression this occurs in every case. Obviously it doesn't. Many diagnoses are relatively straight-forward, and treatment often can be started right away. With difficult-to-diagnose symptoms, though, diligent application of the differential diagnosis process is essential. As new information is acquired, the possibilities must be reviewed regularly. An open mind is an important asset.

Medical Testing: Helpful Friend or Confusing Foe?

Despite major advances in technology, most physicians still operate under a principle instilled during their training days. This principle states the history and physical examination should play major roles in diagnosis; laboratory, X-ray, and other testing servcs only to confirm the clinical impressions.

That's somewhat idealized. Some aspects and functions of the human body are more accurately measured by tests than by examination. For example, chest x-rays can more accurately determine the size of the heart than a physician can by examination. Lab tests are important for finding liver damage, which may not show up on physical exam. The electrical activity of the heart can be studied for extended periods by devices such as a Holter monitor, which may detect intermittent abnormal rhythms not found during regular examinations.

With most lab tests or diagnostic procedures, problems can occur at a number of points. The specimen may be incorrectly collected, improperly handled, or mislabeled. A problem can occur during the testing procedure; the lab personnel may not perform the test correctly or they may be distracted. An incorrect amount of specimen may be used. A slide could be stained improperly. If a technician or physician needs to interpret information at a certain point, errors can occur. Even if the correct result is obtained, information must be accurately transferred to the physician. If a number of tests have been ordered, it's easy to overlook missing results. Unfortunately, test results sometimes are filed before the doctor has a chance to review them.

Considering the possible problems during diagnostic testing, it's surprising the process operates as smoothly as it does. When problems do arise, it's the physician's responsibility to inquire about a missing test result and to question results that seem misleading or that don't jibe with other information.

This returns us to the idea that medical testing is primarily confirmatory, though at times it complements the diagnostic process. Tests should be selected to prove or disprove diagnostic possibilities. If a "shotgun" approach is used, more problems can be created. When a large number of tests are done, the likelihood of encountering at least one abnormal result is high.

A study reported in the British medical journal *Lancet* looked at 200 patients who had one or more abnormal results on a hospital admission biochemical screening.[3] These abnormalities were unexpected and unexplained. When patients were seen again two years later, only three had developed medical conditions that could be related to the previous abnormal test results. If all the abnormal results had been aggressively investigated initially, 98.5 percent of the patients could have been subjected to unnecessary, possibly risky, and expensive tests and treatments.

This raises the question of what "normal range" really means. For many lab tests, the "normal" is a statistical range determined by testing a number of people believed to be normal. A range of values is then created for that test that includes 95 percent of perceived "normal" people. However, even when the result is actually normal for a particular patient, 5 percent of the time it can fall outside this normal range. Interpretation of abnormal results, especially those close to the normal range, requires care, since many of these are probably truly normal.

On the other hand, a result that falls within the normal range isn't always normal. An individual's usual range for any test tends to be much narrower than the normal range for a large group of people. Therefore, a change in a test result for a particular patient, even when "within normal limits," could be significant. This information could be useful, but unfortunately other factors confound such subtle test interpretation. For example, different laboratories, different lab personnel, and different test procedures may have been used, making comparisons difficult.

Some lab tests frequently produce abnormal values, often near the normal range. For example, this is true for some tests used to evaluate collagen-vascular disorders, such as systemic lupus erythematosus (SLE)—a disease notorious for its varied and subtle manifestations. The erythrocyte sedimentation rate and fluorescent antinuclear antibody (FANA) test often show mildly abnormal results. Also, positive FANA tests are more common in older patients. We then need to ask if the result is actually normal or is it a sign of a disease process? Some individuals can have persistently abnormal results without ever developing signs of disease.

Obviously, the responsibility for accurate diagnosis can't be abdicated to medical testing. Heavy reliance on technology won't resolve diagnostic dilemmas. Specific tests should be chosen to answer specific questions, but results must then be cautiously analyzed.

But what if there still isn't an answer? As you probably know, it's possible to go through an exhaustive physical examination and undergo a series of diagnostic tests without discovering a diagnosis. This is frustrating, but it's important to understand that reaching a firm— and correct— diagnosis may require time. And in some cases, no diagnosis can be made.

Nevertheless, progress is possible while diagnoses are being eliminated, new information is acquired, and physical changes are quickly recognized. Knowing certain diagnoses have been excluded is reassuring to both you and your physician.

I think it's sometimes difficult for doctors, including myself, to understand why patients find it easier to accept a formidable diagnosis than no diagnosis at all. Probably only those of you who have been in that situation can fully empathize.

Medical knowledge is incomplete. Potentially risky diagnostic and treatment decisions often must be based on clinical assumptions— made before all the facts are available. Each option has pros and cons that must be carefully weighed. Predicting the future is fraught with miscalculation.

When a medical problem has defied diagnosis, it could be a mistake to narrow the list of possibilities too quickly. "No answer" is usually better than the wrong answer, but this can mean living with uncertainty for a period of time. At this point, the patient can enter a monitoring phase during which periodic re-evaluations or a trial treatment might be appropriate. Alternatively, referral to another physician for a second opinion might be helpful. A psychological or psychiatric evaluation would be a third option.

Raising the idea of psychological assessment can be difficult—for both physician and patient. Although the patient may feel the doctor doesn't believe his or her story, the primary purpose of a psychological or psychiatric exam is to gather additional information. It's not, or at least shouldn't be, an attempt to abandon the patient or transfer care to someone else.

Psychological symptoms in a patient with chronic, troubling, yet undiagnosed symptoms aren't at all unusual. What's difficult is knowing whether the psychological changes are a result of the problem ("secondary" changes, meaning they occurred as a reaction to chronic physical symptoms) or whether they're causing the symptoms (primary).

If a psychologist or psychiatrist can't identify a primary or causative psychological factor, the primary doctor must continue to search for a diagnosis.

Please don't misunderstand what I'm saying. A psychological evaluation is just another medical opinion. It can be correct, but it can also be incorrect. It can't be unconditionally accepted and must be critically reviewed. Still, in the right situations, a mental health assessment can be very valuable. It's important to understand these potential benefits any time such a referral is suggested.

Why Are Certain Diseases So Difficult to Diagnose?

Characteristics of some diseases make them particularly difficult to diagnose. For instance, certain diseases tend to cause fleeting symptoms interspersed with long periods of normal functioning. Others cause symptoms common to many disorders, making definitive diagnosis difficult.

Sometimes in the earliest stages, lab studies tend to be negative, normal, or unreliable. Rare disorders may not be considered unless they have very distinctive signs and symptoms. Unusual symptoms with common diseases can also delay diagnosis. Entirely new disease processes are difficult to diagnose until a good deal of information is gathered and reported.

Among the difficult-to-diagnose illnesses is systemic lupus erythematosus (SLE), in which the patient's immune system forms antibodies against elements of his or her own cells. An internal battle wages, causing varied and sometimes transient symptoms. General problems, such as fatigue or loss of appetite, are common but nonspecific don't speed the diagnosis.

One internal medicine textbook states, "Diagnosis poses little problem if the presentation is relatively acute, with classic symptoms and signs and positive laboratory tests."[4] It goes on to say, "Frequently, however, clinical presentations are atypical or symptoms occur so sporadically as to make diagnosis quite difficult."

Some immunologic antibody test results may be barely outside the normal range, further confusing diagnosis. Under these circumstances, extended, careful observation, often for months or years, is required before the diagnosis can be made with certainty. Common misdiagnoses in the early phases of SLE include rheumatoid arthritis, multiple sclerosis, and depression, among others.

Multiple sclerosis (MS) is similar to SLE in that it's also an autoimmune disease. In this case, the patient's immune system is attacking the myelin sheaths, or insulation, surrounding nerve fibers in the brain and spinal cord. Symptoms vary in type and duration. Although classic clinical definition requires that the patient have had at least two separate episodes involving different neurological symptoms, other clinical courses are possible.

Some patients have a chronic, slowly progressive form that primarily attacks the spinal cord. The classic relapsing and remitting form can later become progressive. MS has certain demographic characteristics, being more common in whites than other races, occurring in significantly higher percentages in northern latitudes in the United States, and most often affecting people between age 20 and 40. Diagnosis may be difficult if the situation doesn't fit the usual guidelines.[5]

Diagnostic testing for MS has become increasingly sophisticated. Magnetic resonance imaging (MRI) can show typical MS lesions, but it doesn't make the diagnosis. There can be other explanations for these lesions. Various other tests have been developed to measure antibody production within the nervous system, but they aren't specific for MS. Other diseases can cause similar abnormalities.

Early in the course of the disease, MS often shows false-normal test results. As the disease becomes more obvious, the likelihood of abnormal, and therefore diagnostically helpful, results increases. Unfortunately, the early phase, when diagnosis is least certain, is also the time when test results are least reliable.

Textbooks still note MS is a clinical diagnosis and warn against overreliance on lab tests. It's also noted that diagnosis can take some time, often "several years between the onset of first symptoms and the confirmed diagnosis of MS."[6]

Autoimmune disorders are by no means the only diseases that confound physicians. A pertinent example is Lyme disease. The first case was reported in the United States in 1969, and the possible range of clinical symptoms was described six years later, in 1975. This infectious disease is caused by a bacteria carried by several ticks and is especially common in areas where those ticks are prevalent.

Signs and symptoms of Lyme disease vary widely. Differential diagnosis includes lupus, MS, and many other diseases. A characteristic rash called erythema chronicum migrans (ECM) is often among the early symptoms. However, the rash can be absent or go unnoticed in 20 percent or more of patients. It's been noted that "diagnostic difficulty arises with early or atypical Lyme disease, when systemic symptoms occur before, or in the absence of, ECM, or when neurologic, cardiac, or arthritis complications occur without a history of ECM."[7]

Although there are several serologic tests for antibodies to Lyme disease bacteria, the reliability and proper interpretation of the results are controversial. Most, but not all, patients with major organ system involvement have positive antibody tests— but so do 10 percent or more of healthy individuals living in tick infested areas.

A positive test, particularly with no history of a rash, may mean that person was exposed to the Lyme disease bacteria but successfully fought off the infection without developing symptoms. Conversely, some persons are diagnosed with Lyme disease based on symptoms and signs, even though they have negative or borderline antibody tests.

New medical problems are identified periodically, with acquired immunodeficiency syndrome (AIDS) being a familiar example. AIDS is caused by a new type of virus, possibly a mutation, and can completely destroy the immune system.

Recently another new medical problem was identified linking L-tryptophan with muscular aching, an increase in white blood cells, and inflammation of muscles. In some cases this disorder has caused death. Until the problem was recognized, L-tryptophan was available in health food stores as a treatment for a number of ills, including insomnia.

Researchers are still debating whether the disorder is caused by L-tryptophan itself or by contaminants found in some products.[8] Until an association was made and reported in the medical literature and popular press, this diagnosis would have been very difficult for physicians seeing only isolated cases. In this situation, prompt and widespread reporting may have saved lives.

Summing Up

Ideally, your relationship with your physician should be satisfying for both of you. As the patient, you need empathy as well as explanations for symptoms and a treatment plan. Your physician wants a satisfied patient, along with the intellectual reward of making an accurate diagnosis. However, when a diagnosis isn't easy, the doctor-patient relationship can fall apart. A patient might question a physician's competence or concern. Even if not questioned, a physician might be frustrated and assume the patient doubts his or her diagnostic skill.

If psychological evaluation is recommended, the patient may think the doctor doesn't believe the symptoms are real. Should the patient refuse to see a psychologist or psychiatrist, that patient might be viewed as inflexible. It's easy to see how lines of communication can break down and the doctor and patient become adversaries. The teamwork needed to diagnose a difficult problem is lost.

No easy answer or formula will eliminate potential problems during medical differential diagnosis. Yet there are steps you can take to improve your chances of obtaining a diagnosis while retaining your psychological health and maintaining the support of family and friends. This book will discuss many of those ideas. However, I would like to leave you with one recommendation I believe crucial.

When dealing with a difficult medical problem, it's important to find a physician who listens to you, is interested in helping you, and allows for dialogue. With mutual respect, confidence will grow and hopefully the diagnosis will be found.

CHAPTER 3

When There Is No Diagnosis: Your Options

W hat do you do when a physician, or a number of physicians, has thoroughly evaluated your complaints and you still don't know what's wrong?

You've been informed that all pertinent tests have been completed, yet no significant clues have turned up. This may be a rather gloomy point. You originally consulted your doctor with the hope that he or she would provide answers about the source of your discomfort and would subsequently provide a treatment plan. No diagnosis means no explanation for the way you feel, no clear-cut treatment options, and no prognosis.

You probably feel worse than ever. You see yourself in a no-win situation. If something had shown up during an exam or on a test, it might not have been good news. On the other hand, it's a bitter disappointment when your symptoms remain and you realize you are no closer to understanding the cause. Rather than feeling comforted, you feel anxious about the possibility of a serious problem being overlooked. You feel depressed about the money you spent on unproductive tests and appointments. And you're uncertain about where to turn next.

When you don't feel well, it's hard to think logically and clearly enough to take charge of your own health care. It would be nice if someone would just tell you what to do. If your condition has persisted for several months you might be bombarded with well-intentioned advice from friends and family members. Some suggest doctors whom they know are excellent diagnosticians and will certainly get to the bottom of your problem. Others advise chiropractors, massive doses of vitamins, faith healers, or touted cure-alls. Some even try to diagnose your problem themselves. They offer so many different alternatives that your head spins. Although you're grateful for their concern, you don't particularly want to try some of the suggestions. On the other hand, you don't want to hurt their feelings or leave them thinking you just don't want to get well.

As long as you are consciously able, you must be responsible for deciding the next step. To start, it's helpful to review your options. You have several: do nothing, adopt a wait-and-see attitude; continue your search by consulting additional doctors; treat symptoms with trial medications or other forms of therapy; or use alternative or nonmedical resources.

Doing Nothing

Your doctor might suggest doing nothing for the time being, other than waiting a specified period of time (days, weeks, or months) to see what happens. If the symptoms begin to improve or clear up on their own during that time and don't return, it's probably not necessary to pursue any further course. Many conditions do, in fact, eventually clear up without specific medical treatment. If the symptoms stay the same or worsen rather than improving over time, the doctor may decide either to repeat some tests or recommend additional tests. With many types of chronic illness, symptoms fluctuate in intensity or come and go completely over periods of months or years. These are referred to as exacerbations and remissions. Your doctor will be interested in seeing any patterns that develop. He or she may suspect a particular disease but not want to verbalize any thoughts until more evidence is available.

Adopting a wait-and-see attitude will be more feasible if your symptoms are not completely disrupting your lifestyle and sleep patterns. If you're able to keep busy, it will be easier to take your mind off your symptoms without the added worries of neglected job and family responsibilities.

Continuing Your Search for a Diagnosis

If your doctor is completely stumped, he or she might feel it is appropriate to get another opinion, possibly from a specialist. If your doctor is a specialist, he or she might refer you to another one— either in the same field or in a completely different area. If your doctor doesn't refer you and you're uncomfortable with the verdict, you need to initiate the idea yourself. A good doctor should not be offended by a request for additional opinions, knowing that someone else may think of something previously over-looked.

Patients often complain that the more doctors they consult the less likely they are to be taken seriously. Unfortunately, as your records are passed along from doctor to doctor, becoming thicker and thicker, you can encounter physicians who don't have the patience to sort through all the information, get to know you as a person, and form personal opinions concerning your condition. Instead they skim the records and rely heavily on the opinions and conclusions of previous doctors. They assume that if several other doctors haven't found an organic cause, there is none. However, not all doctors make these kinds of assumptions. There are many who are sympathetic to patients in difficult-to-diagnose situations.

When the cause of your symptoms is unknown, it's not always clear which type of specialist is most appropriate to see. A list of areas that doctors specialize in is included in Chapter 4. Your current physician also can give you some guidance.

Treating Symptoms in the Absence of a Diagnosis

Whenever possible, try to avoid medication. All drugs (nonprescription included) have the potential for harmful effects. Treating symptoms of unknown etiology (origin) carries the additional risks of masking serious problems or aggravating rather than helping the situation. However, if your symptoms are causing you a great deal of distress, keeping you from functioning, or disrupting your sleep, you and your doctor, in collaboration, might opt for a time-limited trial treatment before you have a definite diagnosis.

If you have significant pain, you want to find the best way to keep your pain manageable without taking unnecessary risks. Your doctor might prescribe analgesics or muscle relaxants to help you sleep at night. Doctors sometimes also prescribe antidepressants because they are believed to be of value in treating some physical ailments by improving sleep, appetite, and energy levels, and raising pain-tolerance levels. Steroids are sometimes used for treating pain if the physician believes an inflammatory disease is at the root, but these are very risky.

Steroids can cause severe mood and personality changes and disrupt the endocrine system. They can also be quite dangerous when patients have an infection— steroids can turn a minor infection into a more serious one and prolong the course of an illness. This risk is well known in the case of tuberculosis; and in the case of Lyme disease, there is some debate that steroids are equally dangerous. Some physicians recommend steroids to assist antibiotic treatment in certain instances; others argue strongly against them because steroids slow down the immune response and can therefore worsen and prolong infection.

If pain or other symptoms become chronic, consider solutions other than medication. Explore using a TENS unit (a small, battery-powered device that provides transcutaneous electrical nerve stimulation), biofeedback, or other relaxation techniques.

Finding the best plan for you often involves a long process of trial and error. Keep in mind that everyone's body responds differently to treatments and medications. Pain management clinics have helped some people develop programs to manage their particular problem.

(See the appendix to Chapter 10 for a more in-depth discussion of TENS, various relaxation techniques, and pain management clinics.)

Seeking Help Through Alternative Forms of Therapy

There are other forms of therapy available beyond the realm of conventional Western medicine that people seek out when in search of diagnoses and relief of symptoms. It is difficult to assess the value of many of these treatments because a certain percentage of people recover or improve spontaneously regardless of treatment. For that matter, with any form of treatment it is difficult to sort out what percentage of a cure is related to the remedy itself, to the placebo effect, or to the body's natural healing mechanisms.

It's extremely important that you approach various options with a degree of caution. Be especially wary of those who claim a particular remedy or procedure will cure every health problem from a sprained ankle to inoperable cancer. Keep in mind that you are much more likely to hear about the successes rather than the failures of any treatment regimen. Whatever plan you embark on, you will want to be certain no serious risks are involved.

Sometimes there may be psychological benefits in just knowing you're doing something, whether or not the program has inherent curative powers. I tried some nonmedical tactics, including taking an assortment of vitamins prescribed by a chiropractor, ingesting a concoction of food-grade hydrogen peroxide (that was short-lived— it tasted awful) provided by a concerned family member, and having friends pray over me. None of these tactics cured me, but they offered hope when I was feeling desperate and kept me hanging in there at a time when I was feeling abandoned by medical doctors who were offering no solutions.

A caring friend prodded me into seeing a chiropractor, who drew blood and cut hair samples to analyze them for vitamin and mineral deficiencies. The chiropractor told me I was low on several and prescribed a list of each to take on a daily basis. Before I purchased them, I showed the list to a physician who was skeptical of their value, but agreed they couldn't do any harm. After a few months of following the prescribed regimen I did start feeling stronger and was functioning better for a time. I'll never know for sure whether the vitamins really worked, if my improvement was partially a placebo effect, or if my condition would have temporarily improved regardless. But I felt better because I was doing something other than lying around feeling miserable and hopeless. The money I spent on the vitamins was probably worth the psychological boost.

By the way, it's probably worth mentioning that, contrary to past beliefs, placebos have been proven to be of value in treating real physical conditions. Scientists have discovered that the positive psychological expectations induced by placebos can lead to an increase in the body's production of endorphins (natural painkillers) and enhance the body's own healing power.[1] Placebos can't be used to determine the difference between real, organic symptoms and those that are "all in the head" because experiments show placebos produce dramatic results even in specific physical problems.[2] Anything that promotes a positive psychological attitude produces positive placebo effects. In the past it was believed people who responded to placebos were neurotic. However, serious research hasn't shown any relationship between personality and responses to placebos.[3]

In my own case, I can't discount the power of love and prayers. I will always be grateful for what faith I had and for the love and prayers offered by many dear friends and family members. Several studies have shown that patients who pray or are prayed for heal faster and have fewer complications.

A double-blind study by Randy Byrd, a cardiologist, on 393 coronary care patients at San Francisco General Hospital showed interesting results. The prayed-for group did statistically better in several ways, including less need for antibiotics, less need for intubation, and lower incidence of pulmonary edema. Neither doctors nor patients were aware of which group was being prayed for.[4]

Positive beliefs and expectations can reduce anxiety levels and aid the healing process by freeing more energy for combatting an illness.

The following section provides a brief overview of the most common alternative therapies available in this country. If you're interested in exploring any of these, you can find more information at your library. Some patients have used these to supplement their medical care, and you might want to discuss them with your physician.

Acupuncture

The use of acupuncture, an ancient Chinese remedy, gained attention in this country in the early 1970s after a well-known *New York Times* reporter underwent an emergency appendectomy during the first official visit of Americans to China after the Communist revolution.[5] On returning to the Western world, the news media proclaimed the message that acupuncture really works. The ensuing public demand prompted several controlled research studies, which have shown that the mechanisms involved in acupuncture are physiological and that positive benefits are not due solely to the power of suggestion.[6]

The most popular use of acupuncture in the United States is actually a nontraditional aspect of the procedure. In Chinese medicine the main purpose of needle insertion procedures are to control energy imbalances. However, most acupuncturists in the U.S. use the needles for pain control. The treatment involves inserting extremely thin needles into various points of the body. The needles are left there awhile, then removed. Modern acupuncturists also sometimes use electrical pulses in their needles to enhance the pain-relieving effect. There is probably some correlation between the effects of the TENS unit and the type of peripheral nerve stimulation that creates an analgesic effect during acupuncture treatments.[7]

Acupuncture is not painful, nor does it draw blood. In fact, most people don't even feel the needles, which are no thicker than a human hair. Each needle has a rounded point that pushes tissues aside without cutting them.

Acupuncture doesn't work for everyone. Dr. Andrew Weil points out in his book *Health and Healing* that many acupuncturists in the United States are unskilled in the identification points and use bizarre needle placements.[8] Licensing requirements vary, with some states requiring acupuncturists to also be physicians.

In many parts of the world, acupuncture is used for anesthesia in surgical procedures, for treatment of chronic pain, and for diseases that damage nerves, causing deafness and paralysis. Considering that acupuncture has virtually no reported side effects, it might not be a bad alternative to taking potentially dangerous drugs to treat symptoms.

Shiatsu

Shiatsu deals with the same types of problems as acupuncture but involves manipulative hand pressure at various points of the body rather than needles.[9] The effects come from stimulating the body by creating additional circulation at pressure points. Circular motions of the thumb and palm induce the increased circulation. Charts provide information for do-it-yourself treatment of nonserious illnesses, including fatigue, backache, and toothaches. Never apply pressure for longer than three seconds in one particular spot on the neck, as injury or death could result.[10] Other areas of the body tolerate five to seven seconds of pressure at a time.

Although it is possible to learn shiatsu by studying books and charts, you should see a professional for long-term chronic conditions. Some experts in this field do work in conjunction with medical doctors.

Chiropractic

Chiropractors use other methods of hand manipulation and stimulation in order to relieve pain. They offer spine adjustment and various massage techniques. Although traditionally sought out for relief of back, arm, and leg pain, many claim the ability to treat and cure a wide variety of ailments through massage, nutrition, and exercise programs.

Chiropractic treatment is based on the theory, originated by Daniel David Palmer in 1895, that nearly all disorders can be attributed to incorrect alignment of bones (referred to as subluxations), with consequent malfunctioning of nerves and muscles throughout the body.

Some people claim relief from back and other body pain and from fatigue and weakness through chiropractors. There are some instances in which chiropractic can be ineffective or worsen conditions, including herniated discs and arthritis.

Dr. Weil notes chiropractic appears to be effective for some patients with acute musculoskeletal problems, such as severe stiff necks and wrenched backs but is probably less successful with chronic back ailments.[11]

Modern chiropractors have split into two groups, referred to as the "mixers" or liberals and the "straights" or traditionalists. The straights only use spinal adjustment and will adjust to treat an enormous array of disorders. The mixers, who constitute the largest group, apply vitamin therapy, mechanical massage, special diets, ultrasound, electrical nerve stimulation, exercise, traction, and other procedures in addition to spinal adjustments. Occasionally chiropractors work in conjunction with medical doctors.

Nutrition Therapy

Chances are good that a medical doctor will not question your eating habits or suggest dietary changes unless you have specific medical conditions such as high cholesterol, ulcers, or gallstones. A doctor is most likely to suggest eliminating food that may be contributing to a health problem rather than the addition of foods or vitamin supplements to your diet to improve your overall health. However, I have noted in recent years that some doctors are getting their toes wet in the area of nutrition and vitamins. My family doctor once recommended stress formula vitamins for repeated yeast infections, and a urologist prescribed vitamin C supplements for chronic interstitial cystitis, a troublesome inflammation of the bladder.

No matter what your condition is, it makes sense to pay some attention to nutrition. Most of us are taught the basics of good nutrition early in our lives (probably in junior high health classes), then store the information in the back of our brains.

From youth onward we race through life skipping meals, stuffing ourselves with junk food at home and at fast-food restaurants, and crash dieting when our weight begins to creep up. Unless we happen to join the ranks of modern health enthusiasts, too many of us don't pay much attention to what we eat as long as it tastes good and satisfies our hunger craving. We don't eat three well-balanced meals a day and we substitute worthless calories for food items that could be providing us with nutrients essential to keeping our bodies healthy and capable of fighting off disease. Not only do many of us deprive our bodies of what they need, sometimes we put in substances that further deplete our system. For instance, smoking and birth control pills, as well as many medications, deplete or inhibit the body's absorption of certain vitamins, one of which is vitamin C. We expect our bodies to continue to function well, regardless of how we take care of them.

It wasn't until after my own body was overtaken by an unrelenting illness that I started paying some attention to how I had been treating it from a nutritional standpoint. For years I had pushed myself to the limit physically. I enjoyed being busy all the time and found I worked better under pressure. That may not have been all bad, but I would also binge on sweets frequently and then counteract any weight gain by skipping meals entircly. When I was in a hurry, it was easier to grab a handful of cookies than to eat something good for me.

There's no guarantee I wouldn't have gotten sick had I been eating well and taking better care of my body, but it makes sense that the body's ability to fight off infection and other disease is enhanced when it has a good supply of ammunition for the fight.

Although it is generally assumed that people in this country don't suffer from vitamin deficiencies, Michael J. Gibney, in *Nutrition, Diet, and Health*, suggests the incidence of deficiencies depends on how you define the concept. "If it means being deficient in, say, thiamine, so as to develop beri-beri, then deficiencies are rare. But if by deficiency you mean an observed dietary intake below the recommended, or a clinical blood analysis outside the normal range, then vitamin deficiencies are not uncommon."[12] Gibney goes on to say the average person eating a mixed diet is not likely to be deficient by either definition. However, those who are elderly, sick, or alcoholic are more likely to be in short supply of needed nutrients.

When you're sick, the body's demand for essential nutrients will increase as your body tries to regain a state of wellness. If your symptoms include digestive problems or loss of appetite, the likelihood of deficiencies will increase further. Many drugs will also contribute to the depletion of needed nutrients.

More and more studies are linking levels of certain vitamins in the blood to the body's ability to fight off cancer and other diseases. There is much evidence that people who eat diets that include plenty of fruits and vegetables, which are high in vitamin A or retinol, are much less likely to develop cancer. Vitamin C is also believed to be strongly connected with the body's ability to fight off infection and disease.

The B vitamins are often referred to as the mood vitamins and are especially prone to depletion during stress, whether from overwork, illness, or pregnancy. Some medications may also induce deficiencies in some of the B vitamins.

It makes sense that any stress on the body, including an illness, will most likely increase the need for many nutrients. Therefore, if you are ill and are unable to maintain a balanced diet containing plenty

of fruits and vegetables, it might not hurt to supplement your diet with at least a daily stress formula
vitamin (which contains additional B vitamins) and
some amount of vitamin C.

However, no one has proven that massive doses of
any vitamin will be beneficial. Gibney emphasizes
that once a requirement has been met, indications
are that more won't help.[13] In a few instances
megadoses may be harmful. An overload of vitamin
A can cause dangerous overflow of free, unbound
retinol into the blood, which has been known to
result in death.[14]

Please note that it is not likely that people who eat
diets rich in fruits and vegetables containing beta-
carotine, the precursor to vitamin A, will experience
any problem with blood levels of vitamin A.[15] Huge
doses of vitamin C can also create problems by
inducing a higher-than-average requirement. People
who have taken megadoses of vitamin C for several
weeks have occasionally developed scurvy when they
stopped taking them.[16]

Determining whether or not you are receiving the
proper amounts of each nutrient can be complex,
and many factors need to be considered. There is
probably no way of measuring precisely the proper
amount for you. But there are certainly connections
between what you put into your body and your
health. It might be helpful to ask yourself the following questions:

- What were your eating habits like before you
  became ill? NOT PICKY,
- Have you been operating under stressful conditions for some time?

- Are you a heavy drinker?
- Do you smoke, take birth control pills, or ingest anything else that might be creating a higher demand for certain vitamins?
- Now that you're ill, what are your eating habits like?   FLUCTUATE, SICK LOOKING AT FOOD.

Although poor nutrition is probably not the entire cause of the health problem you're having, there is a chance it has played some role in the process.

Nutritious diets should contain selections from all the food groups, plenty of fresh fruits and vegetables, and plenty of pure water. Avoiding tobacco and potentially harmful chemicals as much as possible might allow the immune system to fight disease better.

If you're interested in exploring the issue of nutrition further, there are many resources available. Keep in mind, however, that common sense in regard to the amounts of vitamins you consume is a good policy.

A good nutritionist may be able to help you plan a program that is best for you. Homeopathic physicians, chiropractors, and osteopaths who practice in holistic medicine also offer nutritional counseling. You may want to check what credentials they have for claiming the knowledge they do. Even though vitamin enthusiasts often claim nutrition therapy will bring about miracle cures for whatever ails you and will keep you forever healthy, I have known some fanatical vitamin-takers who have succumbed to serious illness. However, providing your body with what it needs to fight back in the face of illness can't hurt, and you will stand a chance of improving your sense of well-being.

Osteopathy

Osteopathy concentrates on manipulative (hand) therapy to treat a wide array of medical problems. It's based on the belief that all parts of the body are interdependent; therefore, all parts of the body need to be treated regardless of the specific location of symptoms.[17] Osteopaths are concerned mainly with the musculoskeletal system, aiming towards proper alignment of the vertebrae and organs, and are also concerned with dietary deficiencies.

Training requirements for an osteopath include the same four years of medical training and the same licensing requirements as other physicians. Currently this is one of the largest of the healing sciences outside the areas of traditional medicine and, according to Thornhill, has "a good track record in helping the sick body to restore good health and smooth functioning without drugs."[18] However, Weil points out that more and more osteopaths are resorting to drugs, surgery, and other traditional methods of treatment and, as a group, they are becoming less distinguishable from regular doctors.[19]

Homeopathy

Established in 1810 by Samuel C. Hahnemann, a German physician, homeopathy is a branch of medicine based on the theory that diseases are cured with substances that produce symptoms similar to those presented by the sick person.[20] Hahnemann discovered that a healthy person who took a small amount of quinine would develop symptoms that mimicked malaria. Since quinine was also effective in treating malaria, he deduced that other illnesses may be cured by taking small amounts of substances that produced similar symptoms. In further experiments, he noted this method often produced an immediate worsening of symptoms, followed by a cure.

Other remedies developed by homeopathic physicians include nitroglycerine for anginal pain and metallic gold for arthritis, both of which are now used by traditional medical doctors as well.[21] About five hundred remedies are commonly used today in homeopathic treatment of disease. The remedies homeopaths use are prepared almost entirely from fresh materials and are prescribed in small doses so as not to act on the tissues or aggravate the condition being treated.

Although few controlled studies of homeopathy exist, a 1980 collaboration between traditional doctors and homeopathic physicians published in the *British Journal of Clinical Pharmacology* reported significant improvement in patients with rheumatoid arthritis when they were treated with homeopathic drugs. [22]

Yoga

Although often associated with eastern religions, yoga in the western world concerns itself primarily with the physical aspect of the being and concentrates on various body postures and exercises to make the body flexible and improve the coordination between mind and body. Although some advocates believe that a variety of ailments can be brought under control by resting different parts of the body consciously and unconsciously, many people in this country use yoga solely as a relaxation technique to help cope with stress or to reduce the intensity of their symptoms.

Holistic Medicine

Holistic medicine incorporates an informal collection of attitudes and practices united by the philosophy that good medical practice must take into account mental and spiritual dimensions, as well as the physical. Advocates also stress health and its maintenance rather than disease and its treatment.

Dr. Weil points out that "all sorts of practices go on under the banner of holistic medicine, some of them quite bizarre." Although he applauds the idea of medical doctors emphasizing nutrition and discouraging the use of medication, he expresses concern over what he often sees as an "uncritical acceptance of unorthodox methods by doctors who call themselves holistic."[23]

It is difficult to assess the value of some treatments, especially the nontraditional ones. Therefore, prudence is important.

In his book *Health and Healing: Understanding Conventional and Alternative Medicine*, Andrew Weil, M.D., provides a thought-provoking exploration of the origins of allopathic (traditional) medicine, homeopathy, osteopathy, chiropractic medicine, faith healing, acupuncture, and other medical practices. Although he is trained in allopathic medicine, he believes that some nontraditional health-care alternatives have a place in treating illness.

Dr. Weil offers information about allopathic and alternative medical practices that can help you make choices about health care. He points out that, although allopathic medicine is the best method he knows for treating acute illnesses and handling medical emergencies, it does have definite shortcomings and problems when it comes to treating chronic illness.

Finding Your Own Answers

It's not likely there will ever be an infallible cure-all that will work on every person and for every medical concern known to human beings. Those who claim to have all the answers and the means to end all human suffering are providing a disservice. However, I do believe hope is an essential ingredient of survival.

Hope is what keeps us going in any adverse situation. In my own case, although some of the healing techniques I tried provided little relief, I consider them to be steps on the way to my actual diagnosis and correct treatment.

You may not always make the right decisions. The important thing is that, as much as possible, you take responsibility for your health care and make some kind of decision. If that doesn't prove effective, review your options again. Whether that decision is to learn to live with your condition as is or to continue to pursue a diagnosis and treatment, it's your body and you need to do what feels most comfortable to you.

Most people do opt to find a physician who is willing to work with them, but some find it helpful to explore other resources.

Joyce Abel, a counselor for people with chronic health problems (see appendix), tells of one patient who solicited her services. The woman was dealing with a nonspecific condition that caused her to have constant diarrhea. The problem was severe enough to prevent her from leading a normal life, but her doctor had told her there was nothing that could be done about it. Joyce referred the woman to a nutritionist who was able to work out a diet plan that reduced the frequency of her diarrhea significantly and allowed her to lead a much more comfortable and productive life.

With or without a diagnosis, over time you will begin to understand your illness better and learn the best ways to manage. If you're fortunate, with time, rest, and possibly some form of therapy, your illness will eventually be resolved so you can concentrate on the more pleasant aspects of your life.

If your symptoms level off after the initial onset and remain fairly consistent, you may gradually learn to adjust to them and structure your activities to accommodate them or compensate for the disabilities caused by them. You can learn your limitations and regain some sense of stability in your life.

If your symptoms steadily worsen over time, your illness will place increasing strain on you and your family. This may indicate a progression of the illness, and in this case the likelihood of diagnosis may increase.

The most demanding scenario may be that in which your symptoms are relapsing or episodic—you fluctuate between feeling relatively well and really sick. This type of illness demands a great deal of accommodation on your part and your family's and requires flexibility in your schedule.

In any event, in order to deal successfully with any ongoing undiagnosed health problem, it will be helpful to develop perseverance, to learn to believe in yourself, to hang on to whatever faith you have, to learn to forgive, and most of all to not give up hope.

CHAPTER 4

Finding the Right Doctor

I attribute my successful management of this illness and immeasurably improved quality of life to finding a physician who consistently respected and believed what I had to say—which is not more than any patient deserves. By working with me, rather than in spite of me, he was able to diagnose and begin to treat my disease.
—Eileen Radziunas[1]

W hen you're coping with a difficult-to-diagnosis illness, it's important to find a doctor willing to work with you on managing symptoms, exploring options, and overseeing treatment—even before any diagnosis is found. That physician plays an important role finding temporary solutions, acting as a liaison to other medical services, and offering reassurance and moral support. Ideally you want a physician who not only has good credentials, but who you trust and feel comfortable with. Although I don't recommend indiscriminate doctor shopping, don't force yourself to continue seeing a doctor who doesn't treat you with respect and dignity and doesn't allow you to make decisions regarding your own health care.

People who have confidence in their physicians do better emotionally and physically. Your goal should

be to find a doctor who is open-minded, compassion-
ate, respectful, and willing to work *with* you.

If your illness is affecting many different organs of
your body, or if doctors are unable to pinpoint the
specific problem area, you may need to consult
several specialists. Lyme disease, lupus, multiple
sclerosis, and many other illnesses affect a number
of different organ systems. I was referred to neurologists when there appeared to be central nervous
system involvement, urologists for bladder symptoms, internists and infectious disease specialists for
infection, skin specialists because of a rash, and, of
course, psychiatrists.

For many years my medical care was complicated by
having an assortment of physicians involved for brief
periods of time. Not many of these specialists com-
municated with each other—or spent much time
communicating with me, for that matter. When I
eventually found one physician I could entrust with
my overall care, including keeping tabs on medications and making referrals, the process went much
smoother, and I felt more confident I was getting the
best care possible.

When care becomes too fragmented, the risk of
medical error increases: tests may be omitted or
unnecessarily repeated, incompatible medications
may be prescribed, or important test results overlooked. Your main doctor (usually called your "primary care" doctor) can be a general practitioner or a
specialist. Some doctors are by nature more in-
trigued by medical mysteries and enjoy the challenge
of medical detective work. Others work better with
patients whose problems are more easily defined.
Maybe your family doctor handles acute and easy-to-

diagnose problems well but doesn't have the disposition for a difficult-to-diagnosis case. You shouldn't worry about upsetting your doctor by requesting other opinions or deciding to seek care elsewhere. Your own health must come first.

Things to Consider When Choosing and Evaluating a Doctor

• Does he or she ask detailed questions about your condition, habits, and lifestyle?

A good doctor will try to uncover any factors that may be contributing to your condition. If your doctor isn't the least bit interested in getting to know more about you or your lifestyle, he or she might miss important clues to the cause or opportunities to discover things that are complicating your condition or increasing the severity of your symptoms.

• Does he or she offer explanations and discuss options with you?

It's important for you to know all the treatment options. Even if you ultimately rely on your physician's judgment, you have a right to have some input in the decision-making process and to explanations as to why the physician believes one alternative is better than another.

• Does he or she give you recommendations or commands?

Doctors should make recommendations based on the facts and their knowledge, but you have the right to decide if you want to follow those recommendations.

• *Does he or she take time to discuss possible side effects of prescribed drugs?*

Problems can arise with any drug. Everyone's body responds differently to a given drug. It's important to be informed of possible complications and of activities or foods you should avoid while taking a drug.

• *Does he or she encourage phone calls if symptoms worsen or new symptoms appear?*

Doctors, like the rest of us, need some time away from the rigors of their work. However, if a doctor isn't concerned enough to be bothered when genuine problems arise, I's find another doctor. Just knowing your doctor doesn't mind an occasional phone call for a legitimate concern will reduce your anxiety.

• *Does your doctor have a colleague who covers problems when he or she isn't available?*

You need someone to consult when side effects occur. If your doctor is going to be away for a time, another doctor should have access to your records and be able to respond to your concerns and questions.

• *Is he or she willing to take time to answer questions and explain medical terms?*

When a diagnosis is elusive, it's especially important for you to be as informed as possible regarding tests, procedures, and treatments offered you.

• *Does he or she show interest in how other family members are responding to your illness and seek input from your spouse?*

When you're dealing with a long-term illness, the way people around you respond to your illness will affect you. If the physician is willing to talk with both you and your spouse, you may draw closer together and eliminate misunderstandings. At times a spouse can contribute valuable information about your condition— something you don't immediately recall or hadn't observed yourself.

• *Does he or she consider making referrals to other doctors who may have more experience or knowledge?*

No doctor is going to have all the knowledge and skill necessary to diagnose and treat every patient for every problem. A good doctor doesn't pretend to have all the answers and values input from other physicians when the answers aren't clear.

• *Does he or she seem sincerely interested in finding the cause of your symptoms?*

Beware of a physician who simply brushes off your questions and concerns with comments such as, "Let me do the worrying," or seems uninterested in exploring all the possibilities thoroughly.

Types of Specialties

Your physician might consider referring you to a number of different medical specialists, depending on your symptoms. The referral can be a one-time event to verify an opinion or secure advice. A specialist might make recommendations to your primary doctor and leave the actual care and administration of tests or treatment in his or her hands. However, in some cases, the tests or treatment will require the specialist's continued involvement. In other instances you might prefer to have the specialist become your primary physician. Specialists are usually more expensive than general practitioners, even for follow-up visits involving brief consultations. However, if you're happier with the care you're receiving, the benefits may outweigh the costs.

If you're interested in seeing a specialist and your doctor has not brought up the idea, ask about the possibility yourself. Some specialists require referrals from other physicians; others are willing to see patients who call in themselves. Early in my illness a nurse friend recommended that I see a neurologist. My doctor hadn't brought it up, so my husband tried to schedule an appointment for me on his own, only to be told I wouldn't be seen without a referral from my regular doctor. We assumed this was true of all neurologists, but several months down the road we were able to arrange an appointment with a different neurologist without any referral.

Following are brief descriptions of the various types of physicians and their areas of expertise.

Allergist: Works with disorders in which the body becomes hypersensitive to particular substances (allergens). Problems may include asthma, hay fever, eczema, and other skin disorders.

Dermatologist: Specializes in diagnosing and treating diseases of the skin.

Geriatrician: Specializes in treating the aged and diseases of the elderly.

Gynecologist: Treats diseases of women, particularly those that affect the reproductive system. Some also care for women during pregnancy.

Hematologist: Specializes in treating diseases of the blood and blood-forming tissues. When they also treat cancer, they are called oncologist-hematologists.

Internist: Covers a range of specialties, including cardiology, endocrinology, gastroenterology, nephrology, and hypertension. An internist may specialize in just one of these areas; subspecialists in internal medicine include:

- **Cardiologist:** Specializes in diagnosing and treating heart problems.

- **Endocrinologist:** Treats metabolic disturbances involving the endocrine glands and their secretion of hormones (for example, thyroid diseases, diabetes, and obesity).

- **Gastroenterologist:** Specializes in diseases of the gastrointestinal organs, which in clude any part of the digestive tract, the liver, biliary tract, and the pancreas.

- **Infectious Disease Specialist:** Deals mainly with bacterial, fungal, and viral illnesses.

- **Nephrologist:** Specializes in kidney diseases.

- **Oncologist:** Specializes in treating cancer; often subdivided into medical, surgical, and radiation specialties.

Neurologist: Specializes in diagnosing and treating diseases of the nervous system, including the brain, spinal cord, and peripheral nerves.

Obstetrician: Cares for women during pregnancy, childbirth, and the period of about six weeks after delivery.

Ophthalmologist: Specializes in diagnosing and treating eye diseases.

Osteopath: Treats a wide array of disorders but concentrates on the musculoskeletal system. Treatment emphasizes manipulation rather than use of prescription drugs.

Orthopedist/Orthopedic Surgeon: Specializes in treating diseases, injuries, and deformities of bones, joints, and surrounding tissues using prescription drugs, surgery, manipulation, traction, or special apparatus.

Otorhinolaryngologist (ENT): Specializes in disorders involving the ear, nose, and throat.

Pediatrician: Treats infants and children, usually up to age 16.

Physiatrist: Specializes in rehabilitative medicine.

Plastic Surgeon: Deals with reconstructing damaged or deformed parts of the body, for example, repairing damage from burns or accidents or correcting congenital defects.

Proctologist: Specializes in colon and rectal disorders.

Psychiatrist: Specializes in diagnosing and treating mental disorders. Psychiatrists are generally trained in diagnosing and treating the psychological consequences of medical diseases as well, both those that occur directly as symptoms of the disease process and those that occur secondarily in reaction to the experience and consequences of being ill. Unlike psychologists, psychiatrists are able to prescribe medications, as well as provide psychotherapy.

Pulmonary Specialist: Treats diseases associated with or affecting the lungs.

Radiologist: Specializes in either diagnosing or treating diseases through radiation, including X rays and radioactive substances.

Rheumatologist: Specializes in diagnosing and managing diseases involving joints, tendons, muscles, and ligaments. Includes various forms of arthritis and other inflammatory (autoimmune) conditions.

Urologist: Specializes in problems of the urinary tract.

There are times, especially in difficult-to-diagnose cases, when the opinion of more than one specialist in a given area might be in order.

Resources for Finding a Doctor

If you have recently moved, aren't happy with your current physician, or simply have never needed to develop a relationship with a physician before, you may want to check with friends, neighbors, or relatives to see if they can suggest good physicians in your area. Keep in mind that people often appreciate different qualities in a physician and you may not be pleased with the way a doctor handles your particular situation. Find out what people like and don't like about the doctor they recommend. Some people are most concerned with a doctor's manner, while others worry more about competence.

The American Academy of Family Physicians provides a free list of family physicians in your area. The address is 1740 West Second Street, Kansas City, Missouri 64114. The phone number if (816) 333-9700.

Your local medical society also can provide information. Although they will not make specific recommendations, discuss competence, or give information about fees, they can provide directories listing physicians in your area, the schools they attended, the places they practiced, their ages, addresses, and telephone numbers.

You may prefer choosing a younger physician who graduated recently. Although a young doctor might not have a great deal of experience, he or she might be more knowledgeable about recent medical discoveries. A younger doctor is also more likely to be in the process of building a practice and more inclined to spend additional time with patients. On the other hand, you may prefer an older physician with more experience who may have encountered patients with similar symptoms.

Annette Thornhill suggests asking members of the medical profession you have contact with who they turn to for their own medical care. She states that, in general, patients seem happier with doctors in group practices. She attributes this to the fact that these physicians stimulate and challenge each other.

This type of practice also makes it easier for your doctor to arrange for someone to fill in when he or she is unavailable.

Whether or not a doctor is affiliated with a research center might also influence the likelihood of your receiving a diagnosis. Research doctors are often interested in cntering patients into specific studies, with stringent criteria for inclusion and exclusion. As a result, criteria for the diagnosis of a disorder will be very strict. Doctors at a research center might send patients away, saying the patients don't have a disease because they don't meet the standard criteria. However, a clinician working out of a private office is more likely to be interested in helping the particular patient and therefore might be more willing to entertain the strong possibility of a diagnosis even if the research criteria haven't been met. It's important to keep in mind that criteria for diagnosis often change, as do the tests that doctors use to identify a disorder.

Other things you may want to consider when choosing a doctor are the types of medical insurance he or she accepts and whether or not the doctor is willing to wait for insurance reimbursement in payment for services. Thornhill suggests the attitudes of people in the office may reflect somewhat the attitude of the doctor. Are they friendly, competent, and respectful toward you?

A common complaint among people I have talked with is they feel worse after a visit to their doctor than they did before they went. This is often the case when they feel the questions they ask are brushed aside and left unanswered, they are made to feel foolish about their concerns, or the doctor seems abrupt, sarcastic, or not genuinely interested in them. With a little persistence, it should be possible for you to find a doctor who makes you feel better, rather than worse, by showing kindness and appropriate concern and expressing empathy toward you in your predicament. It may take a few visits to determine how well you and your doctor are going to interact.

When you have an elusive illness, it's important to find a physician who will evaluate you independently of the opinions of other physicians. Some doctors will not give equal time and attention to a patient who has already consulted a long list of physicians and has not yet received a diagnosis. They might be more skeptical that they can find a physical cause. Although it's best to be as honest as possible, you don't have to pass records on from other physicians when you don't believe the records are accurate or helpful in evaluating your situation.

If you like your doctor, but there's something about the way he or she is handling you case that doesn't set right with you, you may want to discuss it during a visit or drop a note in the mail explaining how you feel about it. The doctor might not be aware of the problem and be perfectly willing to work on correcting it. One man who felt he was rushed through a visit and overcharged put in a complaint and was later granted another office visit for no additional charge. The doctor had had a particularly hectic schedule with unexpected interruptions. Doctors can't know what their patients are upset about if they're not told. Sometimes expressing your concerns in a tactful way will help preserve a valuable relationship with your physician.

If you continually find you're not getting along well with any physician, and they all seem reluctant to handle your care, it may be worthwhile to explore your own attitude and consider the possibility that you're being overly demanding or hostile concerning matters of your care. Finding and maintaining a successful relationship with a physician requires give and take and a certain amount of tolerance and understanding from both parties.

CHAPTER 5

Communicating Your Symptoms and Needs to Your Doctor

"Why can't I find a way to explain myself to the physicians so they can diagnose this illness?" This is a question Eileen Radziunas asked herself again and again as appointment after appointment failed to provide answers to the debilitating pain and fatigue that plagued her for years before she was diagnosed with systemic lupus erythematosus. She began to feel it was somehow her fault that doctors couldn't pinpoint the source of her agony. Her self-confidence plummeted. She became disconcerted with what she saw as her own inadequacy in describing her symptoms.

"I began to take notes on each different type of pain. I was consumed by the idea that explaining my status more clearly was the only hope I had for alleviating the discomfort that had become an everyday fact of life."[1] Eileen continued to make and keep appointments for consultations with physicians but found herself becoming increasingly tense and apprehensive about each visit, worrying that it would just turn out to be another dead end. Yet she was too sick to give up.

Communicating your symptoms to your physician can be one of the most difficult and frustrating aspects of illness. You know that you don't feel right, that you hurt, and that you're not functioning the way you should. But how do you describe what's happening in words that are meaningful to your physician? Doctors told Eileen her complaints didn't make "good medical sense."

We all interpret bodily sensations differently, and patients use different wording to describe a similar pain. People also often have trouble conveying the intensity of their pain. Sometimes you find yourself wishing the physician could temporarily occupy your body and intimately understand your illness– then you wouldn't need to work so hard at describing it. Instead, you fumble along and do the best you can at communicating your concerns and needs under less-than-ideal circumstances.

To complicate the communication problem further, most of us aren't entirely at ease in a medical examination room, anticipating another session of poking, prodding, and questioning. With the apprehension and embarrassment of being told to remove your clothes and perch yourself on an exam table covered only by a flimsy paper gown that rips with the slightest movement, you're at a disadvantage, feeling vulnerable and undignified. By the time you hear the doctor tap on the door, you only wish the ordeal was over. Even if you're usually relaxed and sure of yourself, the setting isn't conducive to straightforward, articulate conversation.

If you've lost a lot of sleep as a result of your symptoms, your nerves may be shot and you might appear overly anxious. It's hard to remember all the things you wanted to mention and all the questions you intended to ask. Too often, following the session, you leave the office worried that you didn't explain yourself very clearly and feeling dissatisfied with the interaction between you and the doctor.

By preparing yourself as much as possible before the visit—whether it's a first time encounter or a follow-up appointment—you help reduce your anxiety level and increase the likelihood of a satisfying encounter with your doctor. Remember to be as specific as possible about every aspect of your condition. Simply announcing that you feel terrible or haven't been yourself lately doesn't give your doctor much to go on. In fact, when you're vague about your symptoms, the doctor is less likely to take your complaints very seriously. The more open and honest you are, and the better account you give of your medical history and current symptoms, the more likely it is that your doctor will be able to help you.

A good start in preparing for your visit might be to write down your impressions of your symptoms at the time they occur. Typically, patients make appointments with their doctors when symptoms are at their worst. Yet if the symptoms aren't of an urgent nature, your appointment will probably be scheduled a few days later. If you're seeing a specialist, it could be several weeks later. By the time your appointment arrives, the symptoms might have changed, lessened in severity, or disappeared. Recalling the intensity or the exact character of the symptoms is more difficult after the fact or between occurrences. Jotting down a few phrases that describe them while you're experiencing them will be helpful. From the time you schedule your appointment until it arrives, continue to take notes on things that come to mind.

Some Questions to Think About Before Your Appointment

• *When did your symptoms first start?*

Be as specific as possible about this. Sometimes you will know the exact day and time you first noticed something amiss. Other times symptoms come on more gradually, and at first you are only vaguely aware of them. Once your symptoms become prominent enough that you're really concerned, you will also be more conscious of other bodily sensations, that may not be related or significant. Mulling this over beforehand will save time during the visit and enable you to give more confident answers.

• *Have you ever experienced similar symptoms in the past?*

If you have, when, under what circumstances, and how do they compare with those you are now experiencing?

• *Have you been using or have you misused any products that could contain toxic substances?*

Consider such things as garden dust, cleaning agents, paints and lacquers, and medications (including over-the-counter products).

• *Are your symptoms constant or fluctuating? Have they become more prominent since the onset or are they decreasing?*

If your doctor is unable to find the cause, document any patterns that appear over time, taking note of anything that seems to aggravate the symptom.

• *How would you describe your discomfort?*

Is the pain sharp or dull, throbbing, shooting, stabbing, or burning? Can you equate it to other pain sensations you've had in the past?

• *Have you noticed any disturbances in bladder or bowel functions or any digestive problems?*

Has there been an increase or decrease in frequency of urination during the day or at night? Have you had diarrhea or been constipated? Do any foods disagree with you?

• *How are the symptoms affecting your quality of life and ability to function?*

Do they keep you awake at night? To what extent have you been able to continue normal daily activities? It's important to convey to the doctor specifically how your current level of functioning is different from the way it was before the symptoms started. Your doctor will find this information very helpful in deciding how the current symptoms represent a serious change from normal.

• *Does anything you do temporarily improve or alleviate the symptoms?*

Note any improvements after eating, changing position, resting, or exercising. For example, abdominal pain caused by some ulcers will usually calm down for awhile after a meal and return once the food is digested. And extremes in temperature can temporarily exaggerate symptoms of multiple sclerosis or other neurological disorders.

• *Has your environment changed in some way?*

Have you moved to a different climate or installed new carpeting or insulation? Some people are much more sensitive than others to certain substances. For instance, a friend of mine began experiencing headaches, chest pain, and shortness of breath after new carpeting was installed in the office where she worked. When she moved to a different office, her symptoms cleared up. Others in the same office were unaffected.

• *Did you take a vacation before the onset of your symptoms?*

Some diseases are more prevalent in certain areas. Finding out what diseases are endemic and what kinds of symptoms they cause might offer clues. For example, if you have spent time at a park or camping in an area endemic for Lyme disease or other insect-borne illnesses, your chances of getting these illnesses will increase.

• *Are your symptoms changing over time?*

Are they staying constant, fluctuating in intensity, or worsening?

• *Have you been running a fever or experiencing chills?*

You might want to monitor your temperature in the morning, afternoon, and evening, as some illnesses produce fluctuating fevers.

• *Have you lost any weight?*

If so, how much, and over what time period?

• *Have any friends or family members experienced similar symptoms?*

If other people in your home or at work are experiencing similar symptoms, this information could provide additional avenues for your doctor to explore— for example, chemical exposure, food contaminants, or contagious diseases.

• *Have you had any recent illnesses or history of trauma?*

Sometimes symptoms can arise after the fact. A car accident or other type of injury can cause symptoms several days or weeks later. Some illnesses can have associated symptoms that linger long after the acute phase of the illness. For example, infectious diseases can initiate depression and lethargy that last for several months.

The more information you can sort out before your appointment, the more efficiently you can spend your time with the doctor. You'll be more prepared to explain to your doctor the various aspects of your condition and the impact it's having on your life. When you sound confident about details, your credibility is enhanced.

Write down any questions you think of beforehand, although you may have additional questions after the doctor announces the verdict.

Some Things You Might Be Interested in Knowing

• People who describe their symptoms too graphically aren't likely to be taken seriously.

People who describe every symptom in a dramatic and emotional fashion are more likely to be considered to have hysterical tendencies. (Note: In the medical context, hysterical refers to emotional instability.)

It's very important to convey symptoms as clearly and accurately as possible, using language that's descriptive, but not overly dramatic. People with psychiatric disorders will sometimes use excessively graphic detail in describing their symptoms. For example, "It feels like someone is taking a electric drill and drilling holes in me with a three-inch bit."

• List-carrying patients are more likely to be considered obsessive, especially if they have a very long and detailed list.

Although informative articles in magazines and other periodicals often recommend bringing a list detailing information about your condition and questions you want to ask, in some cases doing so could encourage the doctor to form some wrong conclusions.

According to Dr. Larrian Gillespie, many physicians have been taught that patients carrying lists are phobic or neurotic. She cites a textbook on diagnosis that says note writing is "almost a sure sign of psychoneurosis."[2] However, she doesn't believe this and points out that this stereotype was debunked by Dr. John F. Burnum in the *New England Journal of Medicine*. Dr. Burnum observed 72 list-writing patients and found them to be mentally stable. Burnum's study showed almost all of the list writers had serious physical disorders. He concluded patients with organic diseases do refer to written notes to convey their story—and not because they are peculiar or crazy.[3]

Lists and diaries can be useful, and physicians should recognize their importance. However, realize some professionals view list-carrying patients in a negative way. Changes in attitudes come slowly. Keeping your list as concise as possible will probably be to your advantage, not only for your credibility but also to ensure that you allow adequate time for your physician to ask questions.

• *Doctors have a tendency to believe that a certain percentage of people will begin to imagine they have symptoms of illnesses they read or hear about.*

Whenever a national magazine publishes an article on a new disease, doctors are bombarded with patients who are worried about contracting it or fear they already have it. Unfortunately, some doctors are quick to make assumptions. Dozens of people have confided to me that, much to their dismay, as soon as they mentioned reading about an illness, the doctor becomes abrupt and sarcastic or informs them they're conjuring up symptoms to fit what they read.

You might have some legitimate thoughts and ideas as to the cause of your symptoms, based on research you've done or on information supplied by friends or family. But it may be best not to suggest at the onset of the visit that you just read about an illness and are wondering if it could be causing your symptoms.

If you want the physician's own unbiased impression, allow him or her to first do a careful evaluation, then form his or her own conclusions. Later, if you don't agree with the verdict or the doctor hasn't considered a possibility you believe important, you might want to initiate the idea by saying something like, "I understand (a particular disease) can cause symptoms like mine. Do you think it's a possibility we should explore?"

If your doctor doesn't feel it's worth looking into, ask why not. If you still aren't satisfied, you may want to consult another physician. It's not at all unusual for several doctors to have widely differing points of view.

• *Having another person with you during the interview might be viewed negatively, especially if he or she dominates the conversation.*

At times it can be reassuring to have your spouse or another person with you in the exam room. If you do, it's important that you speak for yourself as much as possible. If someone else does all the talking for you, your doctor may interpret it as a sign of emotional dependency or weakness and be less inclined to take you seriously.

Preparing for Phone Calls

In the event you need to call your doctor between appointments, it's important to be prepared ahead of time, just as you would for an office visit, so you can explain your concerns as concisely and accurately as possible. Physicians have a limited amount of time to spend on the phone and aren't reimbursed for phone calls. You shouldn't make a habit of calling unless it's really necessary.

When you take time to organize your thoughts beforehand (with the exception of extreme emergencies), you'll be less anxious about the call. Define in your own mind the purpose of the call, including any information you want to convey and questions you need to have answered. Write this down on paper, then keep a pencil and additional paper handy to write down any instructions from the doctor.

If the doctor can't talk to you right away, let the receptionist or nurse know where you can be reached, and ask for an estimated time for the return call. Some doctors take a break in the afternoon to return phone calls. Others wait until the end of the day. If you have some idea of when to expect the call, you won't be on edge wondering when or if he or she will call.

After the Exam

Before leaving the doctor's office, don't be afraid to ask for explanations of anything you don't understand. Also, don't hesitate to ask your doctor to write down any unfamiliar terms. This will be helpful if you want to explore other resources for information on a topic or condition. If the doctor offers a prescription, he or she should inform you of possible side effects and instruct you on how to take it. It might be helpful to repeat in your own words any instructions the doctor gives you to make sure you understand them correctly or to have the doctor provide any information and instructions in writing.

If you're consulting a doctor on a continuing basis about a chronic condition, it might be worthwhile to keep a record of your visits, noting any medications or other treatments that are prescribed. Before the next visit you can review it, see how well you followed the plan, and be able to evaluate the results.

With time and experience your communication skills should improve, and you will probably begin to feel more at ease talking with doctors. Although I felt intimidated for a long time, I eventually became more confident in myself and more comfortable asking for explanations and offering comments and suggestions. With a change in my own manner came a change in the way doctors responded to me. The quality of my encounters with doctors in general improved immeasurably.

In Chapter 7, we'll discuss in more detail what you should know about tests, medications, and your medical records and suggest sources for additional information.

CHAPTER 6

What to Expect from Your Doctor

Life is Short,
the Art long,
Opportunity fleeting,
Experiment treacherous,
Judgment difficult.
—Hippocrates

T he frustration Americans feel toward physicians as a group is undeniable— and almost
universal. In my experience, whenever the subject of
doctors' attitudes or diagnostic skills comes up, I
hear the same complaint: Physicians simply aren't
living up to our expectations. We criticize them for
not being available when we need them, not being
concerned about the whole person, not listening, and
not communicating clearly. We describe them as
arrogant, condescending, money-oriented, judgmen-
tal, and authoritarian.

Although some of these allegations are founded,
obviously, there's another side to the issue. Just as
it's difficult for doctors to put themselves in patients'
shoes, it's equally hard for us to understand how
stressful and painful it is for physicians to fill the
enormously challenging role expected of healers in
our society. Their attitudes and actions are shaped

and influenced by training, daily pressures, and beliefs about what others expect from them.

In his book, *Healing the Wounds*, David Hilfiker provides a remarkably honest look into his life as a physician, describing his agony over not being able to live up to the impossible expectations placed on him. He candidly discusses his own mistakes and the dilemma between his difficulty in admitting and discussing them openly and his need to be healed of the emotional anguish resulting from them. He reminds us physicians are suffering as well as patients, pointing out that many are falling victim to drug addiction, alcoholism, and suicide.

> *American doctors, whether rural family practitioners or high-tech surgeons, face expectations from their patients, from their own profession, and from the society at large that are utterly unrealistic on a day-to-day basis. They are asked to be Renaissance men and women in an age when that is no longer possible; they are expected to be ultimate healers, technological wizards, total authorities. . . Who could live up to such a world of expectations without either crumpling or hiding behind the masks of omniscience and omnipotence?*[1]

A century ago physicians didn't have the same kinds of demands placed on them. Before the discovery of antibiotics and other miracle drugs, cures were not expected. Infant mortality was high, women often died during childbirth, and it wasn't unusual for people to succumb to diseases that are curable today.

In the last fifty years medicine has acquired greater power to diagnose and treat many diseases. Today we're blessed with an impressive assortment of drugs and awe-inspiring advances in technology. Magazines and newspapers are filled with articles promising even better medicines and diagnostic tests. The message is that doctors should have everything they need at their fingertips; if we avail ourselves of their tremendous knowledge and skill, our medical problems will be solved.

We not only expect doctors to have all the right answers, we also expect answers to be quick and easy. We expect physicians to be available at all times, to know everything about the body, and to always be in perfect physical, mental, and emotional health. We expect them to make the right decisions. We expect them to work miracles.

However, the explosion of medical knowledge in recent decades has made the practice of medicine more complex and in many ways even more difficult and stressful.[2] Because medical science is expanding so rapidly, it's not humanly possible for physicians to keep abreast of all the new developments, even within specialties. Many physicians admit feeling inadequate in spite of spending considerable time reading medical journals, attending continuing education courses, and conferring with other specialists.

We have placed doctors on pedestals— surrounded by all those expectations. We tend to forget they're human. They get stressed out. They suffer anxiety, depression, loneliness, and burnout. They inevitably make mistakes, and those mistakes are likely to have profound effects on patients. An unintentional miscalculation or oversight can prolong an illness or diagnosis and cause permanent impairment or even death.

Although physicians suffer emotional consequences of errors, their training discourages discussing their mistakes and fears with anyone.[3] Such feelings often are swept under the rug. By not being able to talk about mistakes or emotions, physicians are cut off from healing. They're unable to ask for forgiveness and therefore receive none.[4] It becomes easier to deny mistakes or blame patients, the people they work with, or the system. Hilfiker reflects the feelings of many colleagues when sharing his own difficulty in dealing with the paradox of being a healer, yet at times doing more harm than good.

The drastic consequences of our mistakes, the repeated opportunities to make them, the uncertainty about our culpability, and the professional denial that mistakes happen all work together to create an intolerable dilemma for the physician. We see the horror of our mistakes, yet we cannot deal with their enormous emotional impact.[5]

In medical school physicians are lectured and drilled on the structure and dynamics of the human body in health and disease. The emphasis is on the diagnosis—finding out which organ has broken down, discovering what caused the breakdown, and determining the prognosis. No wonder physicians are uncomfortable with cases that are difficult to diagnose. They've been indoctrinated with the notion that it's unacceptable to not have solutions. Perhaps because of this mindset, many physicians tend to

adopt a list of catch-all diagnoses where they catego-
rize all the problems that don't seem to fit anywhere
else. It's much easier to attribute elusive symptoms
to a virus, a psychological disorder, or depression
than to search for a solution or provide no answer at
all. To add to his or her own need for closure, the
physician feels pressure because the patient expects
or demands a diagnosis and specific treatment.

Although trends are gradually changing, the develop-
ment of interpersonal skills between doctors and
patients has been virtually ignored in medical training. Such things as understanding the impact of
illness on the life of the patient and understanding
the physician's own emotions and stresses involving
patient care simply were not explored or discussed.
Everyone seemed to assume that, once out of medical school, the necessary skills would develop naturally. Instead, there is much disillusionment, pretense, and a lack of trust between doctors and patients. Bernie Siegel says it eloquently in Peace,
Love & Healing:

> Medical school teaches everything we need to
> know about writing prescriptions, but nothing
> about understanding people. While I don't think
> most physicians are villains, I do think the training
> process of physicians is villainous. . . . Students
> have their natural desire to help people drummed
> out of them by medical school training that, on
> the one hand, has warned them about maintain-
> ing a professional distance from their patients,
> and on the other, has not helped them to deal
> with such difficult problems as how to tell some-
> one they have AIDS or cancer or how to deal with
> the fears that arise within themselves[6]

Pysicians seldom have any formal training in handling difficult-to-diagnose situations. They're taught to focus on diseases rather than on people and are at a loss when they can't find the specific disease, let alone treat it successfully. Their sense of frustration might come through to the patient as abruptness or sarcasm.

What patients often aren't aware of, partly because doctors haven't been open about it, is that the diagnostic process can be incredibly complex, demanding, and uncertain. When a diagnosis is uncertain, how aggressively should treatment of symptoms be pursued? When do you draw the line on expensive and risky tests in trying to determine the cause of symptoms? Many decisions involve risks of increased suffering and death.

Physicians are expected to be competent in many different areas, must accumulate and retain a vast quantity of information, and must be knowledgeable about many technical procedures. They must choose appropriate laboratory and x-ray tests from hundreds of possibilities. Once the information is gathered, they must sort it out and determine what is and isn't significant. There are seldom specific guidelines, nor are there any guarantees that they're doing the right thing.

Physicians have reported situations where they ordered thousands of dollars worth of tests that produced no answers, only to have the patient recover spontaneously after the tests are completed. On the other hand, they may order dozens of tests, yet omit the one that would have solved the puzzle. Doctors often are tormented by whether or not they have made the right decisions. Should they have pursued testing further? Have they already gone too far?

Like everyone else, doctors have bad days and sometimes simply run out of gas. In addition to seeing patients at the clinic and the hospital, they're often on call at home. Many admit to feeling completely drained at times, even when things are relatively quiet and they should feel well rested.

Most physicians go into medicine with the idea of helping humanity. Still, many react to stress and pressure by detaching themselves emotionally from their patients and becoming authoritarian. Some distract themselves by becoming preoccupied with monetary rewards, prestige, and efficiency. It is less stressful, less time-consuming, and more ego-satisfying to deal with patients who have definable illnesses.

When you or someone in your family is ill, you want your doctor to be concerned. It's disappointing when he or she seems aloof or matter-of-fact. However, if your symptoms aren't life-threatening, it may be difficult for the doctor to empathize. Other patients may have more severe problems that require immediate attention, and your situation might not seem serious.

The nature of the doctor-patient relationship encourages physicians to deal with patients as problems to be handled rather than persons in need of care. If your problem doesn't appear as urgent as others, the doctor might not be motivated to show the kind of concern and spend the amount of time you hoped for.

This information isn't intended to discourage those of you suffering from undiagnosed illness. But by understanding the physician's perspective, we as patients might be able to explore ways to encourage them. Maybe they, in turn, will be less inclined to respond in ways that make us feel worse instead of better.

After interviewing a number of physicians personally and having the opportunity to speak on doctor-patient relationships from a patient's perspective, I'm reassured that most doctors aren't close-minded. On the contrary, most are eager to learn how they can better serve their patients. I've had opportunities to speak at medical conferences and have been warmed by the number of physicians who approach me afterward, shaking my hand vigorously and thanking me for telling them, as they say, "things they needed to hear."

What they need to hear is there's so much they can do for patients aside from providing a diagnosis and prognosis or cure. It's human nature to need to feel a sense of accomplishment. Doctors are no exception. They, too, need to feel rewarded for their efforts. And those rewards are above and beyond money. I suspect many physicians don't feel good about charging patients when they feel they haven't helped.

A mutually satisfying doctor-patient relationship is possible with or without a diagnosis. Dr. Witek was enormously helpful to me before my diagnosis, even though he didn't make that diagnosis. He made a favorable impression the first time I met him by simply saying, "This must be terribly frustrating for you. You deserve some answers." Just having a doctor acknowledge it wasn't easy for me to have some nameless affliction was uplifting. And realizing he respected me as a person was a great comfort.

I sensed that my case presented a puzzle Dr. Witek was compelled to solve. Our relationship was probably enhanced, too, by the fact that my own attitudes and expectations had changed during the years I spent dealing with the medical profession in my search for an answer. I was happy to find someone willing to explore treatment options, rather than dictate my medical care. I was more aware of the limitations of medical science, more inclined to demand a role in decision making, and willing to accept responsibility for the consequences of those decisions.

Before my illness, I thought there were definite tests and specific treatments, if not cures, for most illnesses. I believed most medical decisions were based on concrete scientific knowledge. It was basically black and white. Gradually, through experiences and research, I learned how wrong my assumptions were.

I've worked through my anger about the many blunders that occurred during my search for answers. But I still find myself wishing doctors would have taken time to explain what they must have known from the beginning: Medical tests are fallible, and there are simply more unknowns than knowns. That lack of honesty and openness is a source of anguish for the victims of undiagnosed illness. Patients so often feel that if nothing shows up on tests, their symptoms can't be real. Doctors appear to speak with so much certainty about things that are, in fact, uncertain. Hilfiker suggests that much of the dissatisfaction and distrust among patients stems from the fact that the "fundamental issue of the uncertainty of medicine has not been addressed." As a result, both physician and patient are left "feeling misunderstood."[7]

It would be easier on all of us if we would stop the pretense and acknowledge the fact that very often we can't have the answers. Our society categorizes and labels everything to the point that we deny the reality of anything we can't define. Doctors and patients alike need to become more comfortable with the uncertainties of medicine. Even when a diagnosis can be reached, the precise nature of most illnesses is unclear and there might be no cure or definite prognosis.

Doctors' opinions are likely to differ considerably, even in common situations. During the final weeks of my fourth pregnancy I was seeing two different obstetricians who alternated schedules. One week I was told by the first doctor that the baby was positioned head down. The next week, the other doctor emphatically stated the baby was breech, with the head up. The next week, each physician repeated the same information. I knew the baby wasn't turning that much and because each doctor was so convincing, I decided I must be carrying twins. I was almost disappointed when only one baby arrived.

In *Clinical Judgment*, Alvan Feinstein testifies to the many uncertainties of modern medicine.

> *Clinicians are still uncertain about the best means of treatment for even such routine problems as a common cold, a sprained back, a fractured hip, a*

peptic ulcer, a stroke, a myocardial infarction, an obstetrical delivery, or an acute psychiatric depression. . . . At a time of potent drugs and formidable surgery, the exact effects of many therapeutic procedures are dubious and shrouded in dissension.[8]

Doctors sometimes argue that it is better for patients not to be informed of uncertainties— that they really don't want to be told everything and like decisions made for them. However, when doctors aren't completely honest, patients can become disillusioned and lose trust.

What I appreciated most about Dr. Witek was his humbleness and willingness to admit that he didn't have all the answers. He was interested in my ideas and opinions and open to anything that might shed light on the situation. When I told him about the many suggestions and opinions offered by family and friends, he listened and commented with sincerity that maybe one of them eventually would come up with the answer for me.

How refreshing for a doctor to admit that someone outside the profession might be capable of having a bit of worthwhile knowledge about a medical problem. Some go to extremes to protect their authority on health matters. On one visit to her doctor, my mother-in-law mentioned a cold that had lingered for several weeks. She was taken aback when he retorted, "Listen. I'm the doctor. I'll tell you when you have a cold."

Mutual trust is an important key. Once a physician acknowledges limitations, he or she is free to allow more input from the patient and to share decision making. In doing so, both share in the responsibility for mistakes. Who knows? This could even lead to fewer malpractice suits.

Uncertainty is stressful for both doctor and patient, but often we have no choice. When we support each other in coping with uncertainties, we all benefit. Most patients say they wish their doctors would admit they don't know all the answers. Still, a few are upset by their doctor's lack of knowledge. These people need to realize this doesn't mean the doctor is incompetent, superficial, or uncaring. Doctors simply can't be expected to find and fix everything.

In spite of its imperfections, our current medical system has a great deal to offer. Even though many of its fallibilities surfaced during my own struggle, eventually medical researchers discovered how to cure my illness. (It is interesting, though, that Lyme disease became a focus for medical research because of the tenacity of a New England housewife.)

In addition to accepting limitations and uncertainty, we need to learn how to communicate our expectations. In the process, we can find reassurance and hope in knowing we're understood and will not abandon each other. Patients value physicians who demonstrate personal concern and a willingness to listen. These qualities are therapeutic in themselves. Bernie Siegel, in *Peace, Love & Healing*, describes an incident in which he simply went and sat near a seriously ill patient's bed during a brief interlude between surgeries. When he said, "I wish there was something I could do to help you," the patient responded, "You are helping me."[9]

When a doctor is able to exhibit a sense of caring regardless of the nature of the illness, it validates the patient's experience and gives him or her a feeling of self-worth. Sara, a young nurse who suffered severe pain from a form of inflammatory arthritis, reflected on her own prediagnosis stage and the many times doctors made flippant and sarcastic comments. Once, when she complained about pain in her elbow, a doctor remarked, "Oh, you nut!"

This remark and others took their toll on her self-confidence. "I began to feel terribly ashamed that I was taking up all their time with my measly little problems." Much of her pain was in her feet, and she forced herself to try to walk without limping so others wouldn't notice. By the time she was diagnosed with "chronic, progressive, degenerative rheumatoid arthritis," she was told her bones looked like Swiss cheese.

Sara is adjusting to her illness and is off her feet now, working as a nurse consultant and offering empathy to others going through similar traumas. She has managed to keep a sense of humor. During an interview, she alluded to the segment of the Hippocratic oath, *primum non nocere*, which translates to "above all, do no harm." Sara suggests it would help if the phrase be expanded to include "with your mouth." Much of the harm physicians inflict on their patients is through insensitive remarks. The choice of wording by a physician can make an enormous impact, being either devastating or uplifting.

The future appears hopeful as trends seem to be changing. A growing number of doctors and patients are speaking out on the need for changes in the medical evaluation process and more openness in doctor-patient relationships. *Healing the Wounds*, by David Hilfiker; *The Silent World of Doctor and Patient*, by Jay Katz; and *Peace, Love & Healing*, by Bernie Siegel are just a few of the books written by doctors who propose reforms in the current system. There are also many books written by nurses and patients.

Katz discusses at length the idea of informed consent, which was established by judges in the early 1960s with the intention of protecting the patient's right to greater freedom of choice when it comes to medical care and treatment.

No single right decisions exist for how the life of health and illness should be lived. Medical advances have led to a proliferation of treatment options and better understanding of their benefits and risks.

Physicians and patients bring their own vulnerabilities to the decision-making process. Both are authors and victims of their own individual conflicting motivations, interests, and expectations.

Both parties need to relate as equals and unequals. Their equalities and inequalities complement one another. Physicians know more about disease. Patients know more about their own needs. Neither knows at the outset what each can do for the other.[10]

As patients we need to stop expecting doctors to be superhuman. As Barbara Huttmann says in *The Patient's Advocate*, "A physician is a human being—no more no less.... if we have conferred godlike powers on him, which we have, and he has promoted our perception of him as a god-like being, which he has, then we are all responsible."[11]

We need to expect to be treated as intelligent and responsive individuals and to be listened to. We also need to request and expect that doctors be open and honest about the treatments and procedures they offer to us. We need to be informed of the results of all tests. Physicians should respect our right to know possible side effects of treatments and drugs. We should expect to have our questions answered to the best of the physician's ability and be referred to other resources when appropriate. In return, we must respect the doctor's opinion and be willing to listen to ideas and recommendations. We should not try to talk a doctor into procedures and medications he or she doesn't feel comfortable with.

We need to reinforce the idea that doctors can be immensely helpful to us even in difficult-to-diagnose situations. Knowing I had a doctor who was interested in my situation, whom I could call if my symptoms worsened, and who was willing to discuss my concerns was incredibly reassuring.

Bernie Siegel says, "It is important to realize that we will never cure everything. . . . But we can as doctors, as family, and as friends, care for everyone. . . . In that caring true healing will occur— the healing of the spirit and of lives.[12]

CHAPTER 7

Being Your Own Medical Detective

Courtesy, privacy, and information are the three basic rights of all patients and the greatest of these is information.
—*Barbara Huttmann, RN[1]*

A re you a "good" patient? The stereotype that comes to mind is someone who doesn't complain a lot, follows the doctor's orders to the letter, and doesn't ask too many questions. He or she is submissive and conforms to the system. In fact, the word *patient* means to endure suffering without complaining. Unfortunately, the *good* patient runs a risk of being victimized by poor health care.

Many doctors prefer patients who don't make waves— simply because they require less time. Modern clinics and hospitals focus on efficiency. The less time spent with each patient, the more patients processed in a day. The doctor takes charge by telling the patient what to do rather than offering alternatives. He or she brushes off questions and concerns by saying, "Let me do the worrying."

When I questioned one doctor about the risks of a spinal tap, he retorted, "If you are worried about it, then you will probably have problems." Although I was angered by his cockiness, at the time I was too meek to defend my right to know. After the spinal tap I endured an excruciating headache for two weeks. I never reported it to that doctor because I was convinced he wouldn't believe me anyway.

I later learned that a procedure called a blood patch, in which the doctor injects a small amount of the patient's own blood back into the epidural space outside the spinal canal, could have countered the headache. This procedure forms a kind of pressure seal and prevents the cerebrospinal fluid from leaking. Dr. Witek says he has only felt it necessary to do this a few times, but each time it has been very effective in alleviating the headache.

The relatively new concept of informed consent legally requires health-care providers to inform patients of risks involved with medical procedures and of alternatives. Patients are gradually becoming more aggressive, demanding involvement in decisions. Some doctors are beginning to realize that keeping patients in the dark is not in the best interest of either party.

When patients share responsibility for decisions, they are less likely to blame the medical profession when results are not what they hoped for. When patients are aware of details concerning tests and records, they are more likely to catch mistakes that have been overlooked. In either event, the doctor spends more time with the patient initially, but saves time in the long run. Many lawsuits result from a failure to disclose information, including the risks involved in surgeries, the harmful effects of treatments, and an explanation of alternative treatments. Informing patients and allowing them more input in the decision-making process could result in fewer lawsuits, leaving a great deal of time and money to be invested in the more positive aspects of health care.

Some doctors believe that giving patients more information only gives them more to worry about. Although some patients may be upset at learning the risks of surgical procedures, tests, and treatments, according to George J. Annas, who wrote *Judging Medicine*, surveys show that most patients prefer to know, and feel more comfortable when they do.[2]

When you're brave enough to challenge your medical care and demand to be informed, you can be a part of the movement toward changing the image of a good patient to one who is responsible and plays an active rather than passive role in health care.

Being a more active participant in your search for a diagnosis and becoming more informed about the care you are receiving might not make you popular with every doctor, but there are times when doing so can benefit you. Finding out exactly which diseases you have been tested for, what the specific results of those tests were (not just whether they were normal or abnormal), and what's in your medical records and hospital charts could at times spare you grief or speed a diagnosis. It can also provide opportunities for you to clear up errors or misunderstandings. There is no one to whom the information is more vital than yourself; you are paying for all of it, and you have a right to know.

As a patient you do have certain legal rights, but until you assert those rights, they are meaningless. By asserting those rights, I don't mean suing doctors and hospitals for everything that goes awry after the fact, but rather asking to be informed beforehand to assure the best care possible.

In 1973 the American Hospital Association adopted the Patient's Bill of Rights, which is often posted in hospitals and clinics. The original text has been altered in some states to conform with various standards; however, the basic premise is that you as a patient have the right to knowledge concerning your care and to make choices about it.

The following is an example of a Patient's Bill of Rights and a Mental Patient's Rights printed in the appendix of *The Patient's Advocate* by Barbara Huttmann:[3]

A Patient's Bill of Rights

1. The patient has the right to considerate and respectful care.
2. The patient has the right to obtain from his physician complete current information concerning his diagnosis, treatment, and prognosis in terms the patient can be reasonably expected to understand.
3. The patient has the right to receive from his physician information necessary to give informed consent prior to the start of any procedure and/or treatment. Except in emergencies, such information for informed consent should include but not necessarily be limited to the specific procedure and/or treatment, the medically

significant risks involved, and the probable duration of incapacitation.

4. The patient has the right to refuse treatment to the extent permitted by law, and to be informed of the medical consequences of his action.

5. The patient has the right to every consideration of his privacy concerning his own medical care program. Case discussion, consultation, examination, and treatment are confidential and should be conducted discreetly. Those not directly involved in his care must have the permission of the patient to be present.

6. The patient has the right to expect that all communications and records pertaining to his care should be treated as confidential.

7. The patient has the right to expect that within its capacity a hospital must make reasonable response to the request of a patient for service.... When medically permissible a patient may be transferred to another facility only after he has received complete information and explanation concerning the needs for and alternatives to such a transfer.

8. The patient has the right to obtain information as to any relationship of his hospital to other health care and educational institutions insofar as his care is concerned.

9. The patient has the right to be advised if the hospital proposes to engage in or perform human experimentation affecting his care or treatment. The patient has the right to refuse to participate in such research projects.

10. The patient has the right to expect reasonable continuity of care. He has the right to know in advance what appointment times and physicians are available and when. The patient has the right to expect that the hospital will provide a mechanism whereby he is informed by his physician or a delegate of the physician of the patient's continuing health.

—*American Hospital Association*

A Mental Patient's Rights

1. To wear his own clothes; to keep and use his own personal possessions.
2. To have access to individual storage space for his private use.
3. To see visitors each day.
4. To have reasonable access to telephones, both to make and receive confidential calls.
5. To have ready access to letter-writing materials.
6. To refuse shock treatment.
7. To refuse psychosurgery.
8. Other rights, as specified by regulation.

Looking back on my own six-year search for a diagnosis, I can pick out a number of instances in which, had I only been better informed, my saga might have progressed differently. There is even a chance I might have been diagnosed and treated correctly much earlier. One of those instances involved a test for Lyme disease. Early in 1985, during an exacerbation of my symptoms, I was hospitalized for a series of tests. On the final day, I was dressed and ready to be discharged when a lab technician bustled into my room to draw another tube of blood. On my questioning, she reported that the doctor in charge had ordered a test for Lyme disease.

Although it stirred my curiosity, I found that Lyme disease was not even mentioned in the index of our medical guide at home. When I was told a week later that all my tests had come out normal, I promptly dismissed the possibility that I could have this disease, which I assumed was extremely rare. Over the next three years other doctors, on occasion, asked if I had ever been tested for Lyme disease, to which I responded I had.

It was not until late in 1987 that I happened to return to the doctor who had originally ordered the test for Lyme disease. He then informed me of what he had neglected to mention three years earlier— all my blood tests hadn't come back normal. The one for Lyme disease had never come back at all. The lab it had been sent to had responded with a letter saying there was no test available in that state.

Apparently the doctor had not thought it worth mentioning to me or to another doctor who was involved in my case at the time, nor did he consider it worth pursuing by sending a blood sample to an out-of-state lab. When the test was completed, it revealed exposure to the bacteria that causes Lyme disease. I was treated with antibiotics and re- sponded dramatically. My symptoms steadily im- proved over the next two years and today, three years later, I'm energetic and feeling well.

Had I known that Lyme disease was transmitted by a deer tick and that another person who lived in my town had already been diagnosed with it, and had I known my test hadn't been completed, I might have been more persistent in finding a doctor who would have been willing to send a blood sample to an out-of-state lab or to offer a trial treatment of antibiotics.

I've talked with a number of other people who were misinformed about the results of blood tests, which prevented them from receiving care at the time they should have. In other instances doctors have neglected to read the results. One patient, after not receiving word on her Lyme disease test for over a month, finally tracked down the results on her own and learned her test was positive. When she informed her doctor, he was anxious to begin aggressive treatment, but she chose to go elsewhere for her care.

If patients could review the results of their own tests more often, perhaps all doctors would be encouraged to be more careful and thorough, sparing themselves embarrassment and lawsuits.

Doctors' opinions also differ when it comes to interpreting test results. In some cases, borderline tests could be significant, especially when you are exhibiting classical symptoms. Sandy's experience illustrates the importance of not relying too heavily on one doctor's opinion, even when he or she is a specialist.

Sandy was hospitalized for a series of tests after suffering for three weeks with a backache, weak legs, and exhaustion. Two weeks of tests revealed nothing abnormal. However, a 24-hour urinalysis showed levels of aldosterone, a hormone produced by the adrenal glands, at the high end of the normal range. Considering her symptoms, the doctor felt this might be significant and referred her to an endocrinologist, who concluded the results weren't significant. Instead, he suggested her symptoms might be in her head. However, her primary physician wasn't convinced the specialist was right and opted to keep tabs on Sandy's situation. Although a CAT scan performed during hospitalization had revealed nothing, he ordered another one a few months later. This time it showed a small tumor on the adrenal gland. It was surgically removed, and Sandy recovered nicely.

Keeping a list of what you've been tested for, when the test was completed, and what the results were could be useful if you need to consult other doctors in the future. A number of times I was asked if I'd been tested for a particular disorder and had to admit I didn't know— because in most instances I was not told. Even with your records in hand, the new doctor might not review them thoroughly enough to find out what you have been tested for. Tests that are risky, expensive, and time consuming could be unnecessarily repeated.

Other Things You Should Know About Medical Tests

— *No medical test is infallible.*

Few tests give 100 percent proof of the presence or absence of a particular disease. False positives or false negatives can occur. Normal ranges for many tests are approximations, and what's normal for most people might not be normal for everyone. This is discussed in more detail in Chapter 2.

In rare instances machines may be defective or the operator of the machine might not perform the task properly, resulting in faulty results. For instance, electrocardiograms have been incorrectly calibrated or run by unqualified or inexperienced people.

— Laboratory tests can vary from one laboratory to another.

A significant percentage of lab results are inaccurate. According to Annette Thornhill, a government survey of one state's laboratories reported one out of seven tests to be in error or totally unreliable. Sometimes tests are worth repeating by another lab, another doctor, or by yourself.[4]

Not only do some labs have a better overall track record, some might have developed more accurate tests for certain diseases. For instance, tests for Lyme disease are controversial and often one blood sample sent to two different labs will produce con- flicting results. In these instances an institution involved in Lyme disease research is more likely to have good controls and produce more accurate and consistent results.

— Test results are not always evaluated by a physi- cian.

Laboratories outside doctors' offices are supervised and monitored by the government, and testers need to be licensed. However, those in doctors' offices are not monitored and regulated by the government, and at times untrained personnel perform laboratory tests and evaluate test results.[5]

— You can do some tests yourself.

Many pharmaceutical companies are making it possible, in many instances, for people to do some of their own testing, either before they go to a doctor, or afterward. These tests are not intended to take the place of consulting a physician, but to help patients confirm and monitor conditions. For more information on self-administered tests, see the resource list at the end of this section.

— A physician's affiliation with a particular laboratory can limit the places you can have testing done.

Labs associated with research centers are more likely to have better controls and, as mentioned earlier, might have developed more accurate tests for diseases they're currently studying. If you're interested in having a test performed at a lab your physician isn't normally affiliated with, you might request having it sent there and offer to pay any difference in cost.

— Not all abnormal test results are reported by doctors.

A doctor might not report results if they're judged barely outside the normal range and therefore insignificant. In other cases test results are inadvertently filed before the doctor looks at them. If your doctor feels an abnormal test is unimportant, you deserve an explanation as to why.

According to Cathey and Edward Pinckney, who wrote the *Encyclopedia of Medical Tests*, between 25 and 50 percent of tests that turn out to be abnormal are not reported to patients. If you obtain your own copies of test records, you can learn to compare them with the norms.

Types of Diagnostic Tests

X-rays.— With this examination, electromagnetic radiation penetrates the body and provides pictures of internal body structures. Various abnormalities can be detected, including tumors, fluid build-up, and bone changes. Sometimes more tests are required to determine the exact nature of a finding. X-rays should not be overused because of risks with excessive radiation.

Angiography.— An angiogram is an x-ray examination of the blood vessels. A dye is injected into the blood vessels, and a rapid series of x-ray films are taken. Some vessels in the heart, pancreas, or brain can only be seen when they are x-rayed in this manner. Angiographic studies are uncomfortable and expensive. While often helpful to the doctor, angiograms are invasive and are not without serious risk. Therefore, they should be conducted only by reputable and experienced specialists.

CAT Scan.— Computerized Axial Tomography (CAT) is a sophisticated technique that visualizes sections of the body with a special scanner. The scanner feeds information to a computer, which produces a cross-section image of what is "seen." CAT scans are used for detecting masses, tumors, or brain hemorrhages. This is a noninvasive, painless method of examining soft tissues of the body. Sometimes injection of dye is needed to obtain clear images, and some people have allergic reactions to the dye. However, the test is considered relatively safe, and the amount of radiation involved is minimal.

Magnetic Resonance Imaging (MRI)..— MRI relies on magnetic fields associated with nonionizing radiation to produce computerized pictures of soft tissues of the body. It can enable physicians to see delicate nerve fibers in the spinal cord and can differentiate types of brain tissue. Since dense structures do not show up, bones in the skull and vertebral column don't hinder the view. This type of testing is used to detect brain abnormalities, multiple sclerosis, vascular disease, cancer, and other disorders. It is relatively harmless— unless you have metal objects, such as pacemakers or metal joints, that would be drawn to the powerful magnet.

Ultrasound.— Ultrasound is a test based on sound waves, which produce an echo when passed through tissues with varying densities. The echoes are converted into a visual pattern similar to a photograph. This method of viewing the inside of the body is noninvasive and painless.

Oscopy.— Any test with the suffix -oscopy refers to a direct visualization or "looking into" an organ. For instance, a gastroscopy involves inserting a snakelike instrument with a light on one end through the throat and esophagus and into the stomach. The idea is similar to a periscope. Some instruments also allow photographing or obtaining a biopsy of the organ. This is a very direct, but expensive and invasive way to find abnormalities. Some other oscopies are cystoscopy (bladder), bronchoscopy (lung), laparoscopy (abdomen), colonoscopy (colon), and esophagoscopy (esophagus).

Laboratory tests.— Laboratory tests include analysis of stool, sputum, blood, perspiration, tissue, bone marrow, spinal fluid, gastric fluid, cervical secretions, amniotic fluid, pleural fluid, and urine. They are capable of revealing abnormalities at the cellular level of your body. Many laboratory tests involve use of needles. Some, such as a spinal tap to withdraw fluid from the spinal cavity, involve the slight risk of complications, primarily headaches.

Electrocardiography (ECG).— In an ECG electrodes are fastened to the skin of the four limbs and the chest wall and an apparatus called an electrocardiograph records the electrical activity of the heart on a moving paper strip. This test is noninvasive and can aid in the diagnosis of heart disease.

Electroencephalography (EEG).— An EEG records electrical activity from various parts of the brain and converts it into a readable tracing. The recorded pattern indicates the state of consciousness and can detect tumors and other abnormalities, including seizure activity.

Electromyography (EMG).— An EMG records the electrical activity of muscles by means of electrodes inserted into the muscle fibers. This test may be useful in diagnosing muscle and nerve disorders.

Evoked Responses.— Evoked responses are electrophysiological studies of nerve conduction. They measure how fast nerve impulses move from the point of stimulus to the area of the brain that receives them. In diseases such as MS, which involve deterioration of the coating around nerves, the test helps determine which areas of the nervous system are involved, as well as the degree of impairment. Electrodes are placed at specific points and attached to equipment that records the results. These tests are painless.

- **Visual Evoked Response (VER).**— Measures how fast messages travel from the eye to the brain. The subject stares at a television screen with alternating checkerboard patterns.

- **Brainstem Auditory Evoked Response (BAER).**— Measures nerve conduction from the ear to the brainstem. The patient responds to clicking noises of various intensities heard through earphones.

- **Somato-sensory Evoked Response (SSER).**— Checks the rate of nerve conduction from the arms or the legs by applying mild jolts to those areas.

Diagnostic tests can be costly and at times dangerous. Deciding which tests are most appropriate and when to draw the line can be very difficult. Your physician should try to determine which tests will be the most helpful. When the diagnosis is elusive, tests may be ordered primarily to rule out possibilities, rather than to confirm a diagnosis. The doctor needs to use his or her best judgment in order to obtain the necessary information. If he or she is able to avoid going to extremes and subjecting you to serious problems, it will be in your best interests to have the tests done. You should be informed of the known risks and be included in the decision making.

I've already used the terms invasive and noninvasive and maybe I should clarify what they mean. Invasive tests involve entering the skin or body with an instrument and generally run greater risks of complications than noninvasive tests. You will be asked to sign a witnessed consent form for tests with known risks. Noninvasive tests aren't likely to cause harm and don't require signed consent forms. They're also usually less expensive than invasive tests.

Waiting for Test Results

From the patient's perspective, waiting for the results of tests can be one of the most nerve-racking aspects of the diagnostic process. Although results often are available shortly after the test is finished, you often have to wait until your doctor calls you or until the next appointment to learn the results. Technicians or nurses usually won't tell you test results— unless instructed by the doctor to do so. If a series of tests is being done, your doctor will usually wait until all the results are back before giving you any information— unless something very significant or urgent shows up.

With undiagnosed medical problems, you'll probably get used to hearing nothing conclusive has shown up. Because some diseases can take years to show up on diagnostic tests, many will be repeated over time. Doctors also often repeat a positive test to make sure the result wasn't a lab error. If you're anxious to hear the outcome of tests, be sure to ask how soon you'll know the results. Call and ask for a report if you don't hear from them.

Interpretation of test results often varies from doctor to doctor. The findings might only indicate further testing is in order. Your doctor must refer to a list of differential diagnoses (conditions that are capable of causing the symptoms), rule out the ones that don't fit, and zero in on the ones that do. For instance, although most people think of high blood sugar in connection with diabetes, a number of diseases can cause this symptom. By the process of elimination and possible further tests, the doctor usually can zero in on the causes. Test results can be abnormal but still not provide any good clues as to the exact nature of the problem. Medicine is both an art and a science. A doctor's experience, personal expertise, intuitive ability, and knowledge of the patient's medical history all come into play. Some doctors are better diagnosticians than others.

If you are interested in learning more about medical tests or do-it-yourself tests, the following books will be helpful to you: *Encyclopedia of Medical Tests* and the *Patient's Guide to Medical Tests* by Cathey Pinckney and Edward R. Pinckney explain all medical tests that your doctor might order and list normal values for those tests. They also provide information on evaluating the results of tests you do yourself.

The Hospital Experience by Judith Nierenberg provides information on preparing for a test, where it takes place, how long it will take, what the results arc intended to reveal, and what it feels like. She also discusses special care required or problems that can occur following tests.

Concerning Your Medical Records

Unless you specifically request copies of your medical records, chances are you'll never know what's in them. In many cases, there's little reason to obtain this information, and except for lawsuits, I don't know many patients who have asked for copies of their records. However, there are some situations when it may be in your best interest to do so.

When you are chronically ill with an undiagnosed condition and are consulting a number of different physicians, it can be helpful to find out what's in your records before you permit them to be transferred to other physicians. Reviewing your records can provide opportunities to uncover errors and clear up misunderstandings.

I'm speaking mainly from personal experience on this matter. I encountered twenty-nine physicians during my search for a diagnosis. Although I suspected I had been labeled because of a past depressive episode, and I was often left in the dark regarding what a doctor was considering, it never occurred to me to request copies of my medical records. However, more than three years into my saga some early records wound up in my hands enroute to a new clinic and a new doctor.

The specialist I was scheduled to see wanted to review my records before the appointment. Because time didn't permit mailing, I picked them up personally. They were given to me in a sealed envelope, but they were my records and curiosity prompted me to take a look at them. What I found was disturbing, and I proceeded to request copies of my records from other clinics and hospitals as well. Although some were very accurate and well kept, the inaccuracies and poorly kept records of others surprised and angered me.

Past emotional problems had been grossly exaggerated. A one-time short-lived clinical depression that occurred three years before my illness had grown out of proportion to the point one doctor had entered, "This patient has been under psychiatric care for years, but did not admit this to me initially." I never admitted this to him because it wasn't true. Another doctor stated that I had a "strong history of severe somatic complaints with no physiological basis." This information was also unfounded, and there were no past records to support these comments. My husband of eighteen years was as shocked as I was by these entries. One psychological test had disappeared from my records completely, although the interpretations of the test remained.

At times what the doctor told me and what he entered in my records were complete opposites. One doctor suggested to my husband and me that MS was a possibility, and he discussed hospital admission and a trial treatment of cortisone injections. He entered nothing about this in my records. Instead, he stated that he had spent a great deal of time explaining why I couldn't have MS. My husband had been with me at the time, and he and I recalled the conversation the same way. Another doctor highly stressed a psychogenic verdict in our interview but didn't indicate it in his notes. In fact, he entered several physical possibilities, including rare, fatal neurological diseases.

Sometimes records were extremely scanty, and many of the symptoms I complained about (some turned out to be significant) were not mentioned. One doctor entered nothing in my records for six consecutive visits— all of which I was billed for.

I was particularly infuriated by outright contradictions of what I had told one doctor. I remembered the event clearly, as I had gone in for a pre-op physical prior to carpal tunnel surgery. I was having chest pain at the time, but didn't bother to mention it because after two years of almost constant pain, it had become pretty much the norm for me. The doctor, on examining me, noted that I had pleurisy and asked if I'd had a recent cold. I hadn't had a trace of a cold and told him so. He responded, "You *must* have had a cold recently." Again I reinforced that I had not had any cough, congestion, or other sign of one. He entered in my records, "Patient has pleurisy from a recent cold." According to resources I later consulted, the cause of pleurisy should be investigated. Perhaps by attributing mine to a cold, he had an excuse not to pursue the issue further. I had the knifelike pleuritic pains throughout my illness, and other doctors had documented the pleurisy. If anyone had paid attention, the pleurisy could have provided a clue that an infectious disease process was underway.

Entries in my records were not always consistent with test results. According to the expert who interpreted the results of an EMG, there was dramatic impairment of the nerves indicative of severe carpal tunnel syndrome. (This is sometimes consistent with Lyme disease, but in my case might have been work related.) The physician strongly recommended surgery to prevent permanent damage. The degree of discomfort I was experiencing was consistent with the EMG findings. None of this information was relayed to me. My attending general practitioner entered in my records that I may have mild carpal tunnel syndrome. The symptoms I complained of, which included numbness in my hands, significant pain in my arms, difficulty holding onto objects, and inability to sleep without dangling my arms over the bed, were not recorded.

Although I again want to emphasize that the records of some doctors were accurate and well kept, I was upset by the number of physicians who were not honest with me and didn't take my word on even simple aspects of my condition. I couldn't go back and change my records. However, I did have a choice in what I transferred to other doctors. I was able to obtain some admissions of error from doctors, and some wrote letters listing corrections to my records. Seeing my records gave me a pretty clear picture of which doctors I really could trust. There were a few I would not return to unless I had absolutely no other choice.

How to Obtain Your Medical Records

Hospitals and clinics retain medical records for many years, although they don't always welcome requests for copies. In most states, you or someone responsible for you has the right to obtain duplicates of your records. Most states have statutes permitting a judge to order the doctor or hospital to produce all the data they have regarding a patient at the written request of the patient or the patient's guardian. Doctors or hospitals might not be excited about requests for records because they fear an impending lawsuit, or they simply don't want to take time to interpret them for you.

I am personally advising that you request your records only to become better informed. If you have trouble translating what is written, you can look up terms in a medical dictionary. I purchased a paperback medical dictionary, which came in handy for looking up unfamiliar terms used by the doctor. You might also ask a nurse or call the doctor's office for answers to your questions. Because doctors have a limited amount of time, try to rely on other sources of information when possible.

To obtain copies of your records, you must sign a written request form supplied by the hospital or clinic, or you can write a letter requesting release of the records to you. Usually a small fee is required. I found I was able to obtain more complete records from hospitals than clinics. Hospitals sent them directly from the medical records department without notifying the physicians involved at the time. However, when I requested copies from a clinic, the doctor knew of the request and took the opportunity to pull out portions he or she didn't want to release for whatever reason.

In one instance I requested copies of my records from a doctor who scheduled appointments one day a week at a nearby hospital. Although my appointments with him usually took place in the hospital exam room, duplicates of the records were sent back to his clinic. I first requested copies of my records from the clinic. When I realized that entries from three or four visits were missing entirely, I requested copies from the hospital also. From there I obtained the complete records and filled in the gaps.

The records the doctor omitted contained information about test results I had never informed of and comments on the reality of my symptoms, which I'm sure he presumed would not set very well with me. Although other doctors also omitted segments of records, I decided there wasn't much to gain in gathering all the details from briefer visits.

If the doctor or hospital determines it's not in your best interests to have access to your records and withholds them, you will need a lawyer in order to obtain them.

If you don't want any information about your condition given out, you can provide a written order to your doctor, the hospital, or any treatment center, stating that you don't want any information released to others who inquire. Your medical records are supposed to be confidential. However, until and unless you give a written order, information might be passed on confirming you are a patient at a particular facility and what your general condition is.[6]

If you've seen more than one physician from the same clinic and aren't happy with the way you are being treated, you might find it worthwhile to switch clinics entirely. I do believe that at times physicians influence the way their colleagues view your case.

What You Should Know About Medications

During a discussion about medications, a pharmacologist friend commented that one of the first things she was taught concerning drugs is that for every positive effect produced, there will also be a potential for negative effects. That's why it is so important to be informed of side effects and to weigh the odds when taking drugs to treat any kind of medical problem. Today there are thousands of products on the market offering promises to cure and alleviate physical and mental suffering.

Pharmaceutical companies subsidize the curricula of medical schools, and each company spends a huge amount of money to induce physicians to prescribe its own brand of drugs.[7] The incentive for doctors to over-prescribe drugs is powerful. According to Dr. Ivan Illich, dependency on drugs and tranquilizers has risen 290 percent since 1962, and drug companies are making enormous profits from drug sales, with markups as high as 140 times the cost of production.[8]

As patients we need to accept some of the responsibility for the overuse of drugs. In addition to being encouraged by drug companies to prescribe, doctors are pressured by patients who feel better when they leave the office with a prescription in hand. Too often we look at a prescription slip as a sign that we're being taken seriously and that we haven't wasted our time and money on an appointment. Because the desire to be validated is great, the temptation to insist on having medications prescribed can be even higher than normal when you have no diagnosis. I was prescribed over twenty different medications at various times. Many of those weren't helpful. Some produced very serious side effects.

I came to appreciate that, whenever possible, it's better to get along without drugs. I realize there are times when they can't be avoided and times when benefits outweigh risks, but precaution is important. You should understand why you're taking the medication, what it's expected to do, and what the long-term effects might be, so you can weigh the odds and decide if it is worth it.

One urologist prescribed a bladder analgesic for the pain I had with chronic cystitis related to my as-yet-undiagnosed Lyme disease. The medication worked wonderfully at first, and the doctor amiably continued to refill prescriptions at my request. When the effects began to wear off, he prescribed a higher dose. After a few months even the higher dose wasn't helping. I later read a pamphlet issued by the manufacturer and learned that the drug was not intended for long-term use, but only for periods of a few days. There were potential dangers. My doctor never told me this.

Although your doctor should be aware of and inform you of side effects, it isn't feasible for him or her to know every possible side effect or have time to review all this in detail with you. If you're planning to stay on any medication, it will be wise for you to research the probable long-term effects by checking the *Physician's Desk Reference* (PDR) or some other reference book, or by asking your pharmacist for a pamphlet on that particular medication. (I found information in these pamphlets is often more thorough than other sources.)

What your doctor might not know and probably doesn't have time to go into is that many medications disrupt the body's ability to absorb essential nutrients and can disrupt the metabolism in a variety of ways. Even nonprescription drugs can cause problems. For instance, aspirin interferes with the ability to retain vitamin C.[9] Therefore, extended use of large doses can affect the body's ability to fight infection and disease. Knowing these facts might provide incentive for you to try pain-controlling methods other than drugs for ongoing problems. Learning as much as you can about medications makes sense.

When you have an undiagnosed problem, it's even more important that you know which symptoms could be caused by medications, so you can better determine if new symptoms are the result of medication or your condition.

Every person's body responds differently to medication; one person may tolerate a particular drug very well while another person suffers significant side effects. The reason for the vast difference in individual responses to drugs is that we're all biochemically unique. For instance, genetic differences allow some people to safely ingest species of wild mushrooms that would make many other people extremely ill. Dr. Weil points out that biochemical individuality is not emphasized during medical training. Instead, medical students often learn about the effects of drugs "as if they were automatic and invariable" and are later "quite surprised to find that actual patients don't respond as pharmacology tests and pharmaceutical advertising say they should."[10]

Adverse drug reactions range from mild problems, such as hives or drowsiness, to serious damage to organs or even death. Additional hazards arise from combining drugs, as Weil points out in *Health and Healing*: "The average patient in a hospital today is placed on half a dozen drugs simultaneously. How some of these chemicals react with each other is anybody's guess. Moreover, a significant percentage of drug doses in hospitals involve errors: the wrong drug, the wrong patient, the wrong dose, the wrong time."[11] Some medications can cause problems when taken in conjunction with certain foods. It is to your benefit to double check these factors also. Your local pharmacist should be knowledgeable or have access to information regarding this.

Brenda is one patient who benefited from her own investigation in regard to medication. A victim of Addison's disease and diabetes, her adrenal glands fail to produce necessary hormones known as corti-

costeroids. As a result she needs to be on hydrocor-
tisone (a steroid) continuously. However, at one
point her druggist misread her prescription and
supplied her with prednisone, another steroid that
was four times the strength she actually needed.
She realized something was wrong when she started
feeling very ill. She called her doctor who advised
her by phone to double the dosage, which meant she
was then taking eight times the normal dosage of
medication.

Things went from bad to worse. Her blood sugar
levels went sky high, she developed a systemic yeast
infection and acne, she experienced episodes of rage,
and her body swelled until she looked like a football
player. When her doctor saw her, rather than checking her medication, she added additional medication— thyroxine.

By then Brenda was feeling "incredibly miserable"
and having episodes of nausea and vomiting. Again
her doctor prescribed more drugs by phone in attempts to relieve those symptoms. In desperation,
Brenda finally phoned the poison control center and
read through the labels on her assortment of medication.

It was then that she learned she had been given the
wrong steroid ten months earlier, which had started
the cycle that prompted her doctor to prescribe
medication on top of medication to counteract symptoms from her overdose. When the dosage was
properly adjusted, Brenda was once again able to
function well in spite of her illness.

Using Libraries as Sources of Information

If you're interested in doing some of your own research, there are resources available at public libraries and at hospital medical libraries. You can locate literature on specific illnesses that your doctors have mentioned as possibilities, and you can find books that tell about tests or medications. I have talked with many patients who have aided their own diagnosis by becoming more knowledgeable about their condition. Looking up references and cross-referencing sources can help you piece together information that might be helpful. A medical dictionary will provide useful definitions of words you don't understand.

By checking the subject file, you can research specific topics. There may be several disorders listed under "diagnosis" for example, that were written to update doctors' knowledge in specific fields. R. R. Bowker publishes a volume called *Books in Print* (BIP) every year, which lists all books in print in three volumes: the author guide, the title guide, and the subject guide. The subject guide will be useful in finding all the books in print on a topic you would like to research. If your library does not have a particular book you are interested in, a reference librarian might be able to obtain it through an interlibrary loan.

Beyond the public library, you can try a hospital medical library or the biomedical library at a university. Annette Thornhill suggests calling ahead for an appointment so you won't be using books, audiovisual materials, and vertical files at times when they're used heavily by doctors, nurses, and social workers.[12] In the medical library you can find reference books listing specific symptoms. In order to look up symptoms and their possible causes, it's best to be as specific as possible.

In *Ask Your Doctor, Ask Yourself,* Annette Thornhill provides more detailed information regarding the use of public and medical libraries for research.

I've talked with a number of patients whose doctors encouraged them not to research their illnesses even after the diagnosis, saying that doing so might only create more distress and cause them to imagine their symptoms are worse. However, from my own experience and from listening to others, I have come to believe that ignorance only increases the chances of error and causes more problems in the long run. It was a doctor who first decided to test me for Lyme disease, but it was partly due to my own investigation that he proceeded to treat me for it.

It is my hope that, in time, as more patients become actively involved in their medical care, attitudes will change and doctors will welcome active participation from their patients. A good patient should not be expected to be passive, submissive, and unquestioning.

CHAPTER 8

When Your Doctor Suggests a Psychologist or Psychiatrist

I f after an evaluation your physician cannot find a definite cause for your symptoms, he or she might question whether your symptoms could be related to depression, stress, or a deep-seated emotional problem. This can be an awkward point in your relationship. Your doctor might expect you to be pleased that he or she found you in good physical health. If your symptoms are relatively mild and you were mainly seeking reassurance, the announcement can, in fact, come as a relief to you.

However, if your symptoms are having a significant impact on your sense of well-being, and you are convinced it isn't logical for stress to cause the degree of discomfort you are experiencing, the doctor's suggestion that nothing is physically wrong can be disconcerting. Your reaction will involve a complex assortment of feelings:

- Disbelief: How can I be making up all of these symptoms? I can't be that neurotic! They can't possibly be a figment of my imagination.
- Increased anxiety: My own doctor is no longer taking me seriously and is probably going to stop looking for the real cause of my problems. He's giving up on me. What am I going to do now?
- Fear: What if I have something really serious and the doctor is just not finding it?
- Anger: The doctor isn't even giving me enough credit to know the difference between stress symptoms and real illness!
- Humiliation: I don't want to be sick, but I also do not want to be considered unstable. What are people going to think if I tell them my doctor believes this is all in my head? Will my credibility be shot? Will I be labeled a hypochondriac?
- Dismay: If my own doctor doesn't believe I'm really sick, how am I going to explain to my boss that I'm not well enough to return to work? Will my family and friends continue to be so understanding, or will they just think I'm lazy or trying to get attention?
- Self-doubt: Maybe I am a hypochondriac. Maybe I am exaggerating my symptoms. If I am neurotic I would probably be the last to know.
- Guilt: Am I doing this to myself? Do I really want to feel this rotten? What if I have put my family and friends through all this worry and concern for nothing? What if all the money we have spent on office calls and expensive tests has been completely unnecessary?

It's not uncommon for people to respond with a flood of emotions, and it is probably perfectly normal. The emotional impact of the suggestion that your symptoms are psychological can be enormous. You have already been dealing with the frustration and uncertainty of being sick and not knowing why, and now you have a new set of fears and uncertainties to deal with.

However, it is important for you to remain calm and try to keep the situation in proper perspective. Although these reactions and fears are perfectly normal, many of them are unfounded. Your doctor is not necessarily giving up on you or on trying to find the cause of your symptoms. He or she might not consider you mentally unstable. Looking into psychological possibilities is fairly routine and often necessary.

Although physicians, with the exception of psychiatrists, are trained to deal mainly with physical symptoms, it is understood that psychological disorders can produce physical symptoms or at least aggravate them. Furthermore, medical illnesses can have psychiatric effects or consequences. Doctors are taught to consider psychological aspects when evaluating symptoms.

If your doctor has never been in your shoes, it will be difficult for him or her to understand what you are going through emotionally. If you reject a psychological workup too strongly, your doctor could interpret your resistance as a desire to remain sick or suspect that you are afraid to confront deep-seated emotional issues. It is important that you discuss the situation calmly. Coming to a good understanding of your situation will take time, and this could be a crucial point in your relationship with your physician. If the doctor sees that you are open to exploring all the possibilities (even if they seem remote), he or she is more likely to be open to your own thoughts and suggestions. It is possible that a psychiatrist will be able to aid your internist in making a diagnosis and in alleviating some of your distress.

Asking your doctor to explain the reasons for requesting a psychological evaluation is not unreasonable and might be helpful to you. Your doctor's reasons could include any of the following:

- The doctor doesn't have any idea at this point what is causing your symptoms and feels this might provide a better handle on how aggressively to pursue further testing for physical problems. Many high-tech tests are very expensive, and some are dangerous. He or she does not want to subject you to risky procedures unless they are necessary.
- The doctor's gut feeling is that you are exaggerating or overreacting to your symptoms, and he or she would like another opinion.
- The doctor would like to try to uncover any emotional or psychological stresses that may be making your symptoms worse.
- The physician might feel a counselor can help you find ways to cope with the uncertainty of your predicament. It is not uncommon for a doctor to refer a patient with known physical symptoms for counseling if the doctor perceives the patient is having difficulty coping.
- The doctor might not want to deal with your situation any longer or does not want to admit he or she does not know what's wrong. This might be the doctor's way of putting it in someone else's hands.

Some doctors have learned to broach the subject of psychological possibilities more tactfully than others and in ways that make the patient more comfortable with the situation. During one of her seminars, Sefra Pitzele explained that, after feeling humiliated on many occasions by doctors, she finally found one who was very helpful. He told her, "I don't have any idea whether or not your symptoms are in your mind or body, but it doesn't make any difference. You and I will work together until we can get to the bottom of this, and we'll do our best to find ways to help you." His approach was not condescending. He made it clear that her input and ideas would not be discounted and that he was going to stick with her.

Not all doctors create an atmosphere of trust for their patients. Even if your doctor has not, try not to consider his or her suggestion for counseling as an insult or put-down. Your doctor might be trying to cover all the bases and help you in the best way he or she knows how. It can be reassuring to know that many others have received the same suggestion. Lots of people with undiagnosed problems are referred for psychological counseling and experience self-doubt. Gilda Radner, in her book *It's Always Something*, describes being sent to psychiatrists so many times prior to her cancer diagnosis that she dubbed herself the "Queen of Neurotics."

Whether your illness is physical or not, there will be some psychological components. It is impossible to completely separate the mind and the body. Modern science has linked psychological and stress factors to many common diseases including cancer, heart disease, ulcers, and rheumatoid arthritis. Your state of mind will effect your physical well-being and your physical state will affect your emotional well-being. People who have been under prolonged stress are much more likely to experience all types of illnesses, both physical and mental. People who are emotionally distressed or depressed will feel worse physically for a number of reasons. They might not be eating and sleeping properly and can become physically run down. Occasionally severe psychological conflicts have been found to be the cause of significant physical dysfunctions, such as paralysis and blindness.

In his book *Worried Sick*, Arthur J. Barsky lists four things, which he calls amplifiers, that magnify bodily symptoms:[1]

1. Circumstances. How a person experiences a sensation, and whether he or she perceives it at all, depends on the person's circumstances. For instance, soldiers in battle may disregard or be utterly oblivious to severe wounds. An investigation done on soldiers wounded in a World War II battle comparing them to civilians with similar wounds that resulted from surgery revealed that soldiers complained of less pain and used fewer painkillers than their civilian counterparts.

The degree of pain might be determined by what that pain means to the person. During battle a soldier might anticipate, even welcome, a nonfatal wound, as it can result in glory or become a way to escape from the fighting. It also means the soldier still has his life. Whereas, for civilians the trauma is unexpected and unique from what is happening to others around them.[2]

Whether the injury occurs at home or at work and who inflicts the injury will also play a role in its effect. People who experience work-related injuries are less tolerant of the discomfort. If they perceive someone other than themselves as being responsible for an accident or injury, their distress is greater.

2. Beliefs about the cause. When you suspect the cause of your symptoms is serious, the symptoms seem more intense. For example, knowing that the pain in your stomach is simply the result of eating a spicy meal will make the pain easier to tolerate than if you believe it's caused by stomach cancer.

3. Attention paid to symptoms. The more attention you pay to your symptoms, the more intense they will seem. Any kind of distraction will decrease the pain. At night, when there are few distractions, pain is usually much worse.

4. Mood. Any kind of mental discomfort will increase any physical discomfort you are experiencing. Strong emotions produce physiological changes throughout the body that intensify symptoms and cause a lower tolerance to pain.

In addition to the four amplifiers Barsky mentions, *expectations* influence pain tolerance a great deal. If you break an arm by falling from a tree, you expect it to heal in three or four weeks, and you might find it easy to tough out the discomfort. However, if the pain is related to a condition you do not expect will improve and that cannot be medically corrected, you might react very differently.

Whether a problem is acute (of brief duration) or chronic (long term) will affect the patient's attitude. When pain or other symptoms are acute, the patient expects them to go away in a reasonable time and is usually not overly concerned about them. However, a patient who realizes or suspects that the problems are chronic will most likely encounter depression, fear, and anxiety.

When you're sick and don't know why, your symptoms will be affected by all of these factors. The very fact that you don't know the cause makes it much harder to take your focus off them. You probably find yourself paying attention to every detail— attempting to see if a pain is traveling in any direction or increasing in intensity. Very often it is hard not to imagine the worst until you have definite answers.

It can be extremely difficult to untangle the web of the physical and the emotional components of an illness, even for experienced professionals. There are many possibilities to consider: Is the main cause psychological or physical? If it is mainly physical, how much are stress and emotions aggravating the condition? If it is psychological, how do you get to the bottom of it and go about correcting it?

There will probably be no easy answers, and there is plenty of room for error in judgment. It is not uncommon for doctors and psychiatrists to misjudge patients. That fact is apparent by the number of people who spoke up and shared their stories as I was working on this project. Sufferers of real physical illnesses from cancer to infectious hepatitis were initially told there was nothing physically wrong with them. These people included men and women, professionals and nonprofessionals, doctors and nurses, young and old.

Perhaps one of the most extreme examples was that of a nurse who was married to a physician. For over a year doctors were convinced that her bowel problems, which included significant rectal bleeding, were due solely to emotional distress. A flexible sigmoidoscopy (viewing of the inside of the rectum and lower large intestine) had been performed and three consecutive specialists agreed there was no physical reason for her symptoms. They told her it wouldn't be cost effective to do more extensive testing because of her age. (She was 42 and they believed she was too young to have cancer.) Doctors told her repeatedly that she was worrying excessively about insignificant problems, and she became so unsure of herself that she stopped trusting her own instincts and medical background.

"I was at work one day, went in the bathroom and discovered I was hemorrhaging. I told myself I was going to have to quit my job because it must be too stressful." After three more hemorrhaging episodes in the evening of that day, she reported the problem to a doctor, who advised her to go to the emergency room. She was finally diagnosed and began treatment for rectal cancer.

Her main complaint was not so much that the doctors didn't find the problem sooner, but that she was made to feel it was somehow her fault and that she wanted to be sick. It is unfortunate that in many cases, the sufferer of a difficult-to-diagnose illness is made to feel quilty until proven innocent.

Even doctors at well-known clinics do not have all the answers. One woman shared an incident that occurred when she was just starting a family. Several doctors at a prestigious clinic concurred that her symptoms of fatigue, insomnia, and weight loss were due to the stress of being a new mom. Neither she nor her husband could accept that answer and continued to pursue another one. A family doctor finally located a goiter and performed surgery on it. She was soon back to her energetic self.

In light of all the uncertainties, how do you decide what to do when your own doctor suggests stress as a cause of your symptoms or advises you to see a psychiatrist or psychologist? What if you follow through on a consultation and continued therapy or counseling is advised, but you do not feel it is necessary? In the remainder of this chapter we will try to help you make your decisions based on a better understanding of psychological illness in general and we will present a more in-depth discussion of stress and depression in relation to physical symptoms. We will list some types of psychological disorders that manifest themselves with physical symptoms and the criteria for diagnosing those conditions. We will explain why there is often much confusion in diagnosing these conditions and offer suggestions to help you understand your own psychological state.

Looking at Stress Factors

All by itself your undiagnosed illness causes stress by creating physical discomfort, emotional trauma, and spiritual conflicts. In addition, you will continue to encounter other unavoidable external stresses capable of aggravating your symptoms. Any kind of stress will make your condition seem worse. Stress and anxiety can also cause physical symptoms.

When you realize that stress will aggravate your condition, which in turn will cause more stress, it's easy to see how an unpleasant cycle begins and how difficult it can be to determine whether or not stress and anxiety are initiating the symptoms or simply making them worse.

We usually perceive stress as anything that requires increased physical or mental energy. Whether the stress is caused by the physical strain of doing too much yardwork or from the emotional distress of an argument with your spouse, if you are already ill, the effects on your body might be the same. For example, persons with multiple sclerosis can experience a temporary worsening of symptoms from extreme temperature changes, from too much physical work, or from nervousness about a job interview.

Stress-inducing events can include both positive and negative occurrences. The list below shows the top thirty stress-causing events and rates them according to their level of impact. They are taken from the Holmes-Rahe Social Readjustment Rating Scale published in 1967 by two psychiatrists.

For a more complete version of this scale and a discussion of how it works, see the *Journal of Psychosomatic Research*, Vol. 11, 1967, pp. 213-218.

Social Readjustment Rating Scale

Event	Scale of Impact
Death of spouse	100
Divorce	73
Marital separation	65
Jail term	63
Death of close family member	63
Personal injury or illness	53
Marriage	50
Fired at work	47
Marital reconciliation	45
Retirement	45
Change in health of family member	44
Pregnancy	40

Sex difficulties	39
Gain of new family member	39
Business readjustment	38
Change in financial state	38
Death of close friend	37
Change to different line of work	36
Increase in arguments with spouse	35
Large mortgage or loan	31
Foreclosure of mortgage or loan	30
Change in responsibilities at work	29
Son or daughter leaving home	29
Trouble with in-laws	29
Outstanding personal achievement	28
Spouse begins or stops work	26
Begin or end school	26
Change in living conditions	25
Revision of personal habits	20
Trouble with boss	20

The more stress-inducing events that occur within a given period of time, the more likely you are to develop a stress-related health change. On the other hand, when you are ill for a prolonged period, there is an increased likelihood of many of these events, such as divorce, sex difficulties, or change in financial state, occurring.

Aside from developing a serious illness, such as heart disease or rheumatoid arthritis (these and many others are organic diseases, but believed to be strongly associated with stress factors), common stress-related symptoms may include:

• headaches
• neck and lower back pain

- nervous tics
- heart pounding
- high blood pressure (this often has no associated symptoms)
- cramps, diarrhea, and constipation
- stomach pain relieved by food or antacids (peptic ulcer symptoms)
- frequent colds
- irritability, inability to concentrate, frequent accidents, forgetfulness
- insomnia
- decrease in sex urge or impotence

As time goes by, most people become pretty familiar with their own stress-related symptoms. They know that when they push themselves at work, or their kids have been sick for three weeks, they are more likely to develop a migraine headache. They know that when they have been excited or nervous about an upcoming event their stomach will act up between meals. They know that when they have been tense they will get a lecture from their doctor about their blood pressure when they go for a check up.

All of the above symptoms can also be associated with other health problems. The best way to determine whether they are the result of stress is to see if they improve significantly and eventually clear up when you eliminate or minimize the stressors you believe are producing them.

If your symptoms persist or worsen in the apparent absence of increased stress in your life, and if they are not ordinarily directly related to stress, chances are they have some underlying physical cause.

(See the appendix of Chapter 10 for relaxation techniques to reduce the effects of stress.)

Depression and Anxiety—
The Cause or the Result
of Your Symptoms?

If you go to your doctor complaining of vague symptoms such as fatigue, weakness, and lack of appetite, he or she might strongly suspect you are depressed. If the symptoms have not been going on for months and are not severe enough to keep you confined to bed, the doctor might do some routine blood work, but not feel it's necessary to go into extensive testing. However, if your symptoms are accompanied by other physical complaints (for example, pain, nausea, numbness or tingling, bladder or bowel problems) the doctor might want to check into the matter further. If nothing shows up after what he or she feels is an appropriate physical evaluation, the doctor might again discuss the possibility that you are depressed.

It is true that physical symptoms often accompany depression. These are the most common depression-related symptoms:

- changes in sleep pattern (insomnia or excessive sleeping)
- listlessness (low energy levels)
- inability to concentrate
- eating disorders (either lack of appetite or overeating)
- lack of interest in sex or impotence

When physical symptoms are related to depression, they are usually accompanied by mental distress, including feelings of sadness, guilt, hopelessness or worthlessness, and possibly even thoughts of suicide.

There are two basic types of depression:

Endogenous Depression. Endogenous means "from within." This type of depression is usually caused by chemical imbalances within the body. The body requires a delicate balance of hormones and neuro-transmitters to function the way it should. Often when something disrupts that biological balance, the part of the brain that controls mood and personality is adversely affected. That disruption could be caused by the lack of a particular substance in the body, a physical disorder, or a disease (for example, low thyroid or infectious diseases), or a substance put into the body (drugs, prescription or otherwise).

Exogenous Depression. Exogenous means "from outside of." This type of depression is caused prima-rily by events that occur outside of the body. It might be loss of a loved one, loss of a job, or some other significant loss.

It is pretty hard to feel lousy for a long period of time and not be somewhat depressed. It is depressing to be sick. However, if your doctor suggests that de-pression is the cause of your illness, rather than the result, consider the following questions:

• Are you normally a fairly upbeat person but feeling down mainly because your symptoms are disrupt-ing your lifestyle and you are frustrated that you don't know what is causing them?

• Were you physically active and basically happy with your life prior to the onset of your symptoms?

• Had you been getting proper nourishment and rest before you started feeling ill?

- If you are on medication, are you certain the medications are not the cause of your depressive symptoms?

- If you have had some episodes of depression in the past, are you convinced that you never experienced the same type of physical symptoms as you are now?

If you answered yes to these questions, it is not likely that you are having symptoms that are the result of depression, and it might be helpful to explain to your physician why you believe they are not related. If you answered no, it does not mean your symptoms are necessarily the result of depression, but it might be helpful to explore the impact of some of these other factors more carefully.

For a further discussion on depression and coping tips, see Chapter 10.

Psychological Disorders that Cause Physical Symptoms

Almost all physical symptoms have a real physical basis. Even when they are caused by stress, there is a physical reason for the discomfort. For instance, in the case of tension headaches or backaches, the pain is caused by sustained tightness of the muscles. It is important for doctors not to assume that because an evaluation fails to uncover an organic cause for symptoms that one does not exist. Even when a psychological workup reveals conditions conducive to a psychogenic illness, it does not prove that a patient's symptoms are entirely psychological.

Physical disorders for which no physical cause exists are called psychogenic disorders, somatoform illnesses, or somatization disorders. Please note that, although the term *psychosomatic* is used widely to refer to illnesses presumed to have no organic cause, this term correctly applies to physical changes aggravated by psychological factors. The word psychosomatic means "mind-body." Some illnesses, such as ulcers and asthma, are influenced by emotional factors more than others.

True Psychogenic Disorders

Conversion reaction disorder. In a conversion reaction disorder, the ability to function normally is dramatically impaired as a way of compensating for some intense emotion. Conversion reaction symptoms can often be traced to a particular trauma or event in the sufferer's life. The affected person is trying to escape a situation by converting emotional distress to physical symptoms. Although a specific incident can trigger the physical dysfunction, the patient is not intentionally producing the symptoms.

One example of a conversion disorder would be a mother who witnesses the death of her child and is so traumatized by the incident that she goes blind because she is unable to deal with the horror of what she observed. Another would be a soldier whose legs become paralyzed because his fear of going back into the battlefield is more than his psyche can handle. These afflictions are referred to as "hysterical blindness," "hysterical paralysis," and so on because the personality type most likely to develop them is known as histrionic (or hysteric). The diagnosis is made when, after appropriate investigation, no physical cause for the symptoms can be found, and the evaluator is convinced there is a relationship between the symptoms and a psychological stressor. A conversion reaction symptom usually occurs suddenly and resolves a difficult situation for the patient by removing him or her from it.

A skilled therapist might help the patient uncover the real cause, face the problem, and find other ways to cope.

Hypochondriasis. Most people are familiar with the term *hypochondriac*, and we apply the term somewhat loosely to describe constant complainers or people who run to the doctor frequently for apparently trivial matters. Some people tend to talk about their physical problems excessively or exaggerate every ache and pain they have. However, true hypochondriacs are generally consumed with the fear of having a serious disease or believe they already do. They interpret every physical symptom or sensation as a sign of a physical illness and are so involved in their own symptoms that they are unable to think of, or be emotionally involved in, anything else.

The diagnosis is made when appropriate physical evaluation reveals no physical disorder, and the patient's persistent preoccupation with disease is believed to be inappropriate in relation to the symptoms.

Somatization Disorder. The somatization disorder is a condition in which the person has a history of many physical complaints or a belief that he or she is sickly. The person experiences several symptoms from a long list of possible symptoms for which no physical cause is determined, or the complaint or degree of impairment is greater than what would normally be expected under the circumstances.

There are other less specific somatoform disorders. Some are associated with various physical complaints that are in excess of what is considered normal, based on a medical doctor's findings.

Avoiding the Psychogenic Label

Just about anyone who experiences symptoms for which a doctor can find no physical cause is a potential candidate for a psychological label. The diagnosis of psychogenic disorders is highly subjective and based on the assumption that doctors will find a physical cause if one is present. (As we explained in Chapter 2, there are many reasons that a physical cause might not be confirmed for months or even years.) In most instances there is no way of being absolutely certain of a psychological diagnosis.

Many diseases, such as collagen diseases, multiple sclerosis, Lyme disease, and chronic fatigue syndrome, can produce a wide array of symptoms, which are bizarre and fluctuating. One doctor told me early in my illness that I had "too many symptoms"; therefore, I needed a psychiatrist. Later I discovered every symptom I had at the time— chest pain, chills, weakness, numb sensations, head pain, a constant urge to void, low back pain, and loss of appetite— were typical of Lyme disease. When my doctor could not tie them to an illness he was familiar with, he discounted them completely. In other cases, more than one physical problem might be present at the same time, causing confusion and misunderstanding.

Often a psychological diagnosis relies heavily on the fact that an "appropriate" physical examination reveals no physical cause. What is considered appropriate varies a great deal from doctor to doctor. One doctor might not consider more tests appropriate, while another one does. Even if several doctors agree that every possible test has been done, the cause could be one that current tests cannot detect.

Other diagnostic criteria include vague concepts, such as physical complaints being "in excess" of what they should be for the physical findings. It is difficult for a doctor or psychologist to know for sure that the complaints are too extreme. Every person has a different tolerance level for pain, and opinions vary greatly among doctors as to what they consider excessive. In some cases there is more to the patient's problem than the medical exam(s) have revealed.

For thirteen years Jane consulted doctors from a local medical clinic concerning severe abdominal pain, which on more than one occasion landed her in the hospital. None of the available doctors were able to find a reason for the pain. When she finally consulted a specialist in another city, he discovered extensive endometriosis (a condition in which the uterine lining grows outside of the uterus and often causes pelvic adhesions). Surgery freed her of the previously debilitating episodes of pain.

Gilbert was another person whose pain was judged to be excessive for the physical findings. Severe pain in his leg prevented him from working at his job, which required being on his feet all day. When doctors could find nothing amiss, they accused him of just being lazy and wanting an excuse not to work. Gilbert's self-esteem plummeted, and he became despondent. Eventually, his wife coaxed him to find a doctor who would listen. The source of his anguish turned out to be a severely deteriorated hip joint due to rheumatoid arthritis. His pain was located in his leg, which confused his previous doctors. They simply had been looking in the wrong place.

The quality of Gilbert's life improved immensely following hip replacement surgery. The stories that have been related to me are endless, but these examples underscore the need for doctors to give their patients more credit for knowing when something is wrong with their bodies.

The term *preoccupied* is also used frequently in conjunction with psychological illness. Doctors use it rather carelessly. When I obtained copies of my own medical records, I was not pleased to find that one doctor had written that I was preoccupied with having MS.

As I recalled, I had asked questions about it on more than one occasion because a doctor had suggested it as a possible cause for my symptoms. I was trying to understand what was happening to my body. I don't believe I was preoccupied with MS. At the time I *was* preoccupied with finding a cause for my symptoms. For four months they had been disrupting my life. I believe anyone would be intent on finding answers under those circumstances.

The important thing is that both you and your doctor keep an open mind and remain willing to explore all the possibilities, both psychological and physical. Although some doctors are quick to slap labels on people, there are also prudent doctors who don't make rash judgments.

It's probably not unreasonable for your doctor to expect you to have at least one or two consultations with a psychiatrist or medical psychologist if it appears your symptoms are going to be a continuing problem and there are no clear answers. Your compliance might reassure him or her that you are willing to explore every possible angle and that you really want to get better.

A good psychiatric consultant would hopefully be able to recognize patterns of mental disorders, and if you were to consult one, might be able to determine whether or not your symptoms are likely to have a psychological cause.

Several months into my illness, a doctor referred me to a medical psychologist. After a few one-to-one sessions, the psychologist concluded I was not the type of person who was likely to come up with a somatoform illness, and she did not feel that further counseling was necessary. Unfortunately, the doctor who valued her advice enough to refer me to her discounted her evaluation. However, it was helpful to me to have an expert reaffirm that psychotherapy was not the answer to my problems.

If a psychological evaluation shows you are not likely to come up with a somatoform illness, it could encourage your doctor to explore other options further. If the results are not clear-cut, or if you are having trouble dealing with the uncertainty of your predicament, you might try counseling awhile. A professional could help you sort out the psychological and physical components of your illness. However, the key to uncovering psychological causes for any problem lies within you. A skilled therapist can only offer guidance and encouragement.

To help evaluate your own mental state, ask yourself the following questions:

- Have I been afraid of becoming ill for quite some time, or have I worried excessively about every ache and pain even though I am functioning fairly well? Do I immediately assume that every bodily sensation is signaling some serious disease?

- Have I been struggling with an issue I do not want to face?

- Are there advantages to my remaining sick? Are they standing in the way of my striving to get better?

- Am I having a difficult time coping and finding no support from family members and friends?

- Are family members and friends encouraging me to get counseling?

- Am I so depressed I feel unsure I can go on much longer?

If you answered yes to any of these questions, you might want to seriously consider seeking a counselor you feel comfortable with. Remember that just because one therapist is unable to help doesn't mean another will not be able to. If you are on medication for depression or anxiety, you need to be under the care of a medical doctor. Psychiatrists are medical doctors with additional training in treating mental illness. Psychologists are not medical doctors and cannot prescribe medication.

If you don't feel comfortable with a psychiatrist or psychologist after several visits, and you feel you are not making progress, it is best to find another one. This may have nothing to do with the counselor's qualifications. The two of you might simply not be a good match.

When I was struggling with depression, a friend recommended a psychologist. After four sessions we both realized we weren't getting anywhere and both decided I needed to try something different. I was the one who suggested we discontinue, but he seemed relieved and was willing to help me find someone else. A good counselor will understand it often takes the right combination of people for therapy to be effective and will not be offended by your decision to try another source.

After exploring every option, you might be convinced your symptoms have a physical cause. Although you may not be able to immediately convince everyone else, try not to make that your main focus. Your goal should be to be as well as possible.

Concentrate on what does help, whether it's counseling, taking care of yourself by resting and eating right, eliminating as much stress as possible, finding a doctor you trust and work with, or all of these.

Appendix to Chapter 8

Psychological Testing and the MMPI

The most commonly used psychological tests in medical settings fall into two broad categories: tests of intellectual function and personality inventories. Tests of intellect (including so-called IQ tests) are used when there is concern about how the human brain is functioning. Although they have other applications, these tests can evaluate the results of a trauma to the head or a disease that affects brain tissue (for example, a stroke). Intellect tests measure word comprehension, reasoning, hand-eye coordination, memory, and a number of other abilities.

Personality testing in medical settings is more controversial, and probably more threatening to the patient with an undiagnosed illness. While there are many types of personality tests, the Minnesota Multiphasic Personality Inventory (MMPI) is by far the most commonly used instrument. In 1989 a revised version of the test, the MMPI-2, was published. The test consists of 567 true-false questions. The MMPI measures a wide range of psychological characteristics, including potentially transitory emotional states (for example, depression, anxiety), as well as more enduring traits, such as shyness.

Although many of the test questions seem strange to the person taking the MMPI for the first time, the test developers used sound, scientific principles. Briefly, when a patient takes the test, his or her answers are statistically compared with groups of subjects who have either a specific psychological diagnosis, or possess a certain psychological trait or characteristic. When a patient scores high on a particular MMPI scale, it is possible (but not certain) that the patient possesses the trait that scale measures.

In the hands of a qualified interpreter, the MMPI can be uncanny in its ability to describe the type of behavior and stress-coping style of the person taking the test. However, by itself, the MMPI can be quite weak in predicting a patient's psychological diagnosis— particularly in medical settings. Ideally, the test should be part of a more comprehensive evaluation, including a clinical interview, by a qualified psychologist.

Probably the most serious difficulty with the MMPI is not its scientific merit, but the way in which people use it. Often, it is administered when the physician is unable to find a medical cause for the patient's physical complaints. Frequently, the patient regards the test as an accusation that "it's all in your head." This problem is compounded when the administrators don't share the results with the patient, thereby adding mystery and mistrust to the patient's experience with the test.

Even more disturbing is that the persons who interpret the test are often inadequately trained for the MMPI. The test results are plotted on a graph that appears deceptively easy to interpret— and "a little knowledge" can result in an interpretation that is greviously in error. Often a computer interpretation ignores important demographic factors such as age or race or important current circumstances like the death of a loved one.

We offer the following suggestions in the event that you are asked to take the MMPI or some similar test.

Don't be afraid to ask your doctor why he or she wants you to take the test. This question can lead to a much-needed discussion of where you are in the diagnostic process. Depending on the nature of your doctor's concerns, you might prefer that a qualified psychologist or psychiatrist evaluate you, and let that professional decide what tests are appropriate.

If you take a medical test, you have a right to have your doctor explain the results. This same principle applies to psychological tests. Generally, it's best to have a psychologist interpret the results. Make sure, however, that the psychologist is qualified with the MMPI and has specific skills for interpreting the test in medical, as well as mental, health settings.

A good interpretation will include a discussion of your personal strengths, as well as weaknesses. A good test interpretation might also leave you with some ideas for beginning to confronting any problems that show up on the test.

CHAPTER 9

Believing in Yourself

I will never forget the tremendous sense of release when I finally stopped feeling I had to prove anything to anyone, and I knew without doubt I did not want or need to be sick. Before that I spent years questioning my sanity, wondering if I really was fabricating or exaggerating my symptoms for some twisted personal gain. I had been fighting feelings of guilt and worrying that my family and friends would give up on me. Because of my insecurity, I felt I needed to prove to the doctors, to everyone around me, and even to myself that my illness was real.

Ironically, it took a psychotic episode triggered by a prescription drug, two suicide attempts, and a month-long stay in a psychiatric ward before I started believing in myself. I came home after that hospital stay devoid of any emotion but fear, feeling abandoned by God. My ego was shattered. My only prayer for a long time was that I would die before I attempted suicide again because I didn't want to put my family through any more grief. And yet, it was because of that episode, during which every ounce of my credibility had been stripped away, that I reached a point where it no longer mattered what anyone else believed about me. I came to value my faith in God and my belief in myself more than the opinions of others. In the end my faith was strengthened, I became confident in myself, and I learned to trust my own instincts.

So many others have shared with me their anguish over not being believed and their own struggles with self-doubt. When there are no explanations for your symptoms, it is easy for your self-confidence to erode. Even those who have not been told by doctors that their illness is psychological admit to questioning the reality of it when no cause is found. I believe self-doubt and the consequent belief that you need to prove the reality of your illness in order to receive help places more emotional strain on the sufferer than does any other aspect of coping with undiagnosed illness.

Although the physical disabilities associated with lupus can be overwhelming, the lingering emotional scars from my long search for a diagnosis are far more devastating, and perhaps irreparable. The humiliation and self-doubt I felt from not being believed—for such a long time, by so many key people—have been shattering to my self-confidence. This loss of trust has actually been the most destructive element of the illness. I felt ignored and pacified by condescending physicians who undermined my intelligence and questioned my

*sanity. They were obviously in a far better position
than I to call the shots, and influenced each other
repeatedly in the way my case was handled.*
                                        —Eileen Radziunas

Human beings have a need to be validated. One man
suffered from strange symptoms including seizures,
smelling odors that were not there, narcolepsy, and
memory loss for several months before doctors ac-
knowledged his complaints weren't a figment of his
imagination. He vowed to his wife he would never
complain again if he could only find proof there was
a physical cause for his symptoms. She reported
that, from the time he received his diagnosis of a
brain tumor until he died nine months later, he kept
that promise.

When you realize that doctors are doubting you, it's
not unusual to become fearful and angry. When you
suspect family and friends no longer take you seriously, you feel rejected and hurt. Fear, anger, hurt,
and a sense of rejection become obstacles to wellness
in themselves.

When people doubt you, it's easy to start believing
that if you could only prove your symptoms are real
you will receive the help you need and your situation
will improve. In reality, when your efforts do not
work, the problem is compounded. I have talked
with others who say they were so angry about being
discredited that they did not want their symptoms to
go away until they could prove there was a real
physical cause. Their need for validation was so
great, and their aversion to being labeled a hypochondriac so strong, that those feelings overcame
their desire for wellness. I have to admit that there

were times when I too feared that my anger and hurt were standing in the way of my wanting to be 100 percent well.

I realize now I often forced myself to keep my emotions in check, hoping to avoid being further labeled as hypochondriac, neurotic, or hysterical. I felt I had to be stoic or "look good" in order to get help. During one particular visit, I remember listening serenely while a doctor explained his personal perspective of my condition and belief that I most likely needed a psychiatrist. I calmly agreed to set up an appointment with one and left the office poised and in control. However, within seconds after my husband and I drove out of the parking lot, I began sobbing uncontrollably. While in the office I had managed to hold back an enormous amount of fear, anger, and frustration.

I was fortunate to have many supportive friends during my sick years. Although several doctors questioned the reality of my illness, only one friend expressed doubt that my illness had a physiological basis. It hurt. For a long time it gnawed at me. How could she doubt my credibility when we had been close friends? It created a rift in our friendship. Whenever I was around her, I tensed up and found myself on the defensive. My symptoms often acted up more when she was around. I then worried that she was right after all. My self-doubt increased. Was I just doing this for attention? I realize now that my tension around her created emotional stress, aggravating any neurological effects of the Lyme disease. It became a vicious cycle.

Although my husband was generally supportive, as the illness dragged on I sensed he too had his times of doubt. After all, the doctors could find nothing concrete, and they told him so many different things. I knew he was as confused, uncertain, and tired of the whole thing as I was, but it hurt when he became abrupt or sarcastic regarding my symptoms. I worried we were being driven apart by my illness.

I became afraid to be completely honest about my symptoms or my reactions to them. Worrying about whether doctors would take me seriously increased my anxiety about each office visit. My concern that friends and family members would stop believing in me created awkwardness in my personal relationships. I found myself trying to sort out the most believable aspects of my illness and only talking about what I thought would not hurt my credibility. For instance, the fact that my chorea (repetitive, uncontrollable body movement) was often more pronounced when I was in public was disturbing to me because I was afraid it might be interpreted as a desire to attract attention. I was relieved when Dr. Witek explained that most movement disorders are aggravated by the stress of being in public and subside in the privacy of your own home.

Once I started to believe in myself, my true feelings could surface, and I was able to begin to respond to them in a constructive way. When I stopped worrying so much about what everyone else thought, I had more energy for positive things. The quality of many friendships improved, and I began to feel less intimidated about my encounters with physicians.

How do you start believing in yourself in the face of all the uncertainties of undiagnosed illness? A first step is to face the fact there are no guarantees that anyone will believe you, and there is probably little you can do to convince people if they don't. The answer to whether or not your symptoms are the result of a psychological or an organic problem lies within yourself. Ask yourself, "What's really the most important thing to me?" When you can honestly answer that question by saying, "My one and only goal is to be as well as possible and to live as full and productive a life as possible," you can begin to trust your own instincts about what your body is telling you. It will be easier to shift your goals and redirect your energy from proving your illness is real to living the best life you can in spite of your circumstances.

When I was able to stop focusing on my own feelings of rejection and fear and began to concentrate on coping with my illness, my sense of well-being improved. I searched my soul and learned just how much I wanted to be healthy. Yet I was powerless to change my circumstances or anyone else's opinion. I found a sense of inner peace and realized my ability to find joy in life in spite of them.

Although the love and support of my family and friends remained very important to me, I knew that if necessary I could somehow make it without them. I stopped worrying about what to tell and what not to tell doctors concerning my symptoms. I told them exactly what was happening. Whether they discounted those symptoms or not was up to them. I knew I was doing my part, and I would continue to do the best I could in spite of them. I also found the courage to stick up for my rights. When I discovered discrepancies in my medical records, I confronted the doctors and requested they make amends. I learned to ask for help when I needed it and to refuse help graciously when I did not. On either count I stopped feeling guilty about it.

Only *you* know how sick you are and what you are really capable of doing. When you learn to believe in yourself you will feel more confident about taking charge of your health care and finding the resources you need. You will be able to come to terms with your illness, confront and resolve your anger and fear, and stop questioning yourself. Use the energy you gain for taking care of yourself, healing emotional wounds, and offering love and inspiration to others.

CHAPTER 10

Learning to Live with Uncertainty

"I learned that it is possible to create light and sound and order within us no matter what calamity may befall us in the outer world."

—Helen Keller

T here is no magic formula for attaining the emotional healing and spiritual peace so many people have found in the midst of adversity. For some it comes gradually, and for others it comes quite suddenly and unexpectedly. But no matter how it comes, those who have experienced it verify it is worth striving for and that it can happen regardless of outward circumstances.

Corrie Ten Boom, a Dutch woman, found light and hope during a gruesome imprisonment in Ravensbruck, a World War II German concentration camp. Lil Gibsen, a victim of multiple sclerosis, found a life filled with joy even though her illness robbed her of the ability to get out of bed or even feed and dress herself. Job, in the Old Testament of the Bible, found spiritual enlightenment in the midst of tremendous personal loss and physical pain. I found comfort, renewed faith, and a sense of purpose while

I was still dealing with the uncertainties of an undiagnosed illness. I believe all of these things are possible for you, too, once you reach a point of acceptance.

However, on the way to acceptance you might, as most who suffer misfortune, need to muddle through several other not-so-pleasant states of mind. Elisabeth Kubler-Ross, in her book *On Death and Dying*, describes the emotional aspects of terminal illness in five stages: denial and isolation, anger, bargaining, depression, and acceptance. Experts now recognize these five emotions as normal reactions to any significant loss.

For those with chronic illness, it's not realistic to expect to progress in an orderly fashion from denial through depression, neatly resolving each stage and never having to face them again once the final stage of acceptance arrives. Everyone will experience these emotions differently, and as your illness changes over time you will find yourself repeating the grieving process. Some of these emotions will occur simultaneously or in a different order. Nevertheless, taking a look at the emotional stages of grief as they relate to you and your undiagnosed condition can help you to understand and deal with them.

Anxiety and fear are two emotions not listed within the context of the grieving process, but those who suffer undiagnosed conditions frequently mention these two, so I would like to add them to the list for my discussion.

The losses any ongoing illness creates can be multiple— loss of a sense of well-being, loss of employment, loss of ability to participate in familiar pastimes and hobbies, loss of social life, loss of future plans, and loss of a sense of control. When the illness remains undiagnosed, there is also the loss of certainty about the future. There is no prognosis. You do not know how permanent your losses are, nor do you have any idea of how severe they may become.

Because of the nature of undiagnosed illness, the grieving process seems especially complicated. You might have trouble identifying the stages, let alone getting through them. After all, how do you deny something that's vague and uncertain? Where do you direct your anger when you don't know who or what is responsible for your problems? How do you face and overcome your fear when you don't know what it is you are fearing? How can you move ahead to acceptance until you know what it is you are accepting? It's easy to get hung up on bargaining and depression, to continually tell yourself, "If only the doctor could give me some idea what's wrong with me, I could begin to deal with this." When no answers come, your sense of security and self-worth continue to decline.

It is common for those who are diagnosed with a serious chronic illness to go through a period when the illness dominates their thinking. No matter what they do, they remain preoccupied with the illness and what it's doing or will do to their body. They find it difficult to focus on anything else. Ideally, with time, the illness gradually fades into a position of less importance. It becomes just one of the many facets of their lives. However, as long as the illness remains unknown, the preoccupation phase seems to drag on endlessly.

Even though it's difficult, reaching a point of acceptance with your undiagnosed illness is possible and essential to your peace of mind and ability to live a full life in spite of your health problems. If you remain forever caught up in your symptoms and finding a cause for them, opportunities for growth and happiness will slip by. Life is too short to spend all your energy and time pursuing what you might never attain.

Acceptance, however, does not mean giving up all hope of having an answer, nor does it mean you won't continue to pursue reasonable possibilities when opportunities arise. It does not mean you will never feel any traces of anger, fear, or depression. It does mean that once you and your health-care providers are convinced you have explored all viable avenues, you must face the possibility that you may never have a name for your illness and that you must find ways of effectively managing your emotions.

People often say they discover happiness when they accept the fact they can't change their circumstances. Rather than despairing over their lot, they become in tune with a power beyond themselves and within themselves that is greater than the disorder in their outer world. This power is frequently referred to as God.

Sorting Through Your Emotions

Denial

At least a brief period of denial is likely to transpire whenever you are confronted with a significant trauma or loss. The reality of the situation just doesn't sink in immediately. The denial stage can be compared to the time immediately following a severe injury in which the victim feels little or no physical pain. Scientists have attributed this phenomenon to the brain's release of extra endorphins during extremely stressful situations. In the same sense, the person who learns he or she has a life-threatening or crippling illness, might experience emotional numbness for a time— a sense of unreality or that the situation isn't really very bad. For instance, a person might take the verdict of terminal cancer calmly, even cheerfully, at first and feel confident about being able to cope. But with time to reflect on the seriousness of the situation, composure breaks down, making way for other emotions— fear, anger, bargaining, and depression.

When your illness has no name there seems to be nothing to rest on. You may find yourself continually vacillating between denial that you are sick and fear that there is something very seriously wrong with you. You find yourself completely focused on your body even when your symptoms are better, as you try to assess the severity and the reality of your health problems.

Somewhere along the line you need to affirm that, for whatever reason, you are no longer as healthy as you once were, that you have certain limitations, that your lifestyle has changed, and that your relationships have changed, at least to some degree, as a result of your illness. Once you are able to acknowledge these facts, you can begin to sort out and work with your other emotions.

Anger

Many of us were indoctrinated early on with the notion that anger is a negative emotion and should not be expressed. Society taught us that to do so was a sign of immaturity or rudeness. Religion said it was sinful. Perhaps that's why it took me a long time to recognize my own anger and convince myself it was not only appropriate to be angry, but that my emotional well-being depended on my acknowledging and expressing that anger.

Anger is normal and necessary and is not a negative emotion in itself. When expressed appropriately it can be therapeutic and powerfully motivating. When suppressed, it can result in depression or uncontrolled outbursts that inflict emotional or physical harm on others. It can also make you physically sicker than you already are. In *Why Do Christians Break Down?*, hospital chaplain William A. Miller identifies anger as the emotion people have the hardest time acknowledging. "It is the feeling people believe they must stifle more than any other feeling (even sex), and which when repressed or suppressed seems to cause more trouble than any other."[1] When we express our anger in constructive ways, we defuse its destructive power.

Sorting out your anger during the prediagnosis stage will be a challenge. First of all you need to determine with whom and what you are angry. Next you need to evaluate your anger and decide whether or not it is justified. Finally, you must find ways to express it that won't cause you further distress by undermining valuable relationships with family members, friends, and caregivers.

To help you find the sources of your anger, ask yourself these questions:

- Are you angry with the medical profession for not diagnosing you or for the way they have treated you?
- Are you angry with your spouse for not believing you and giving you the support you need?
- Are you angry with your friends for deserting you?
- Are you angry with yourself for your weakness and inability to cope?
- Are you angry with God for letting you down?
- Are you angry with your sickness and the frustration and pain it is causing you?

Anger can serve more than one useful purpose. It can compel you to keep plugging away and find positive aspects of your illness. It can help you conquer pain and live a productive life. It can drive you to find good health-care providers and additional resources to help you cope. It can open doors to better communication with your family and friends.

It is important to realize, however, that whenever anger is directed toward a person, impulsive expression can be more destructive than constructive. It is better to think before you act and make sure you are reacting reasonably so you can express your anger in positive ways.

When you are angry with the medical profession. Sufferers of difficult-to-diagnose illness very often harbor a great deal of resentment toward physicians and need little prompting to go into a tirade about the shortcomings of the medical profession. Some are angry with doctors for failing to find the cause c their problems. More often they say they are angr

because they feel they have been treated disrespect-
fully. One woman who called me was so hostile
toward the entire medical profession that she became
upset with me for telling her I believed there were
some good physicians out there.

Occasionally patients have told me about losing their
tempers in a doctor's office. One man became infuriated and began to shout at his doctor, making such
a scene that he was escorted out of the office and
asked not to return. Another woman impulsively
slapped a physician who told her he didn't believe
she was really sick. However, it seems most patients
complain bitterly to just about everyone— except the
doctor.

Although I, too, was angry at physicians about the
way they handled my case, it took me a long time to
admit it. My anger was overpowered by feelings of
intimidation. I felt I needed to be polite and passive
in the doctors' presence or they might abandon me.

Before choosing a plan of action for dealing with your
anger, it's important to first consider whether you
are directing anger appropriately. If your doctor
honestly believes he or she has done everything
possible, it's not reasonable for you to be bitter
because of his or her inability to help you. You have
the option of seeking help through a different doctor
or other resources. However, if you have legitimate
complaints about careless or insensitive treatment, it
might help to take some kind of action to vent your
frustration. Writing letters explaining why you're
unhappy and talking with clinic managers or patient
advocates in a hospital are possibilities. Direct your
serious concerns about medical mistreatment to your
state board of medical examiners or to the office of

health facility complaints. Remember that with a little tact you are more likely to be listened to and respected than if you go on a rampage. It isn't to your benefit to alienate yourself from the medical profession.

Four years into my illness I was finally able to acknowledge my anger. At that time I had the opportunity to review medical records and discover many discrepancies. When I realized these had been passed from doctor to doctor for a number of years and probably colored the way many of them viewed me, I was outraged. I had a gut feeling I'd been judged unfairly, and when I saw exaggerations in black and white, I could no longer suppress the anger.

I wrote a letter and later phoned the doctor who had originally entered a great deal of false information and let him know I was upset. I knew I was justified and had evidence to back up my accusations. I think he was quite surprised at first because I had never shown any signs of aggressiveness before. The telephone call was productive in that the doctor apologized and agreed to add my letter to my records along with a signed statement from him verifying it was a much truer account of my medical history than he had entered previously. Later he confided he had learned from my case, and it influenced the manner in which he handled future patients. Becoming angry gave me the courage to speak up for myself, which affected all my dealings with doctors from that point on.

Part of my motivation for writing my first book also stemmed from my anger and disillusionment over the way my case had been handled. I felt compelled to make others aware of how emotionally devastating undiagnosed illness can be and how easy it is for doctors to misjudge patients. At the time I started writing my story, my physical condition was worsening and I couldn't help wondering whether I was heading for full-time invalidism. My desire to put my story in writing gave me added fuel to prevent the illness from getting the best of me. Writing was tremendously therapeutic.

I believe much of the anger patients harbor toward physicians is justified. Yet I feel it's important not to create an us-against-them line of thinking. Along with the expression of anger over the negative things should come understanding and gratitude for the dedication, positive contributions, and accomplishments of many medical doctors and researchers.

When you're angry with your spouse or other loved ones. When it comes to those you love, your hurt over the way they respond to your illness is likely to come out in the form of anger. If they seem aloof, hostile, or doubtful that you are as sick as you claim to be, it is painful. Understand that they are also grieving over the changes in your relationship and are probably as confused as you are about the lack of a diagnosis. Everyone might be feeling angry about the situation, and it is important to discuss those feelings with each other. If you really do care about each other, it is important to reinforce that and establish your intention to stick this out together. You feel like the victim, but so are the other members of the family. During those times when you lash out angrily, try to talk it over after you calm down. Explore where that anger is coming from. All of you are angry at the illness, and sometimes that anger will wind up being directed at each other.

In a situation where you feel the illness is creating a rift, it might be helpful to seek counseling. Sometimes a third party can offer insight, draw out your true feelings, and help you find appropriate ways to express that anger.

Talking with other families in similar situations also is helpful. I am involved in a Lyme disease support group that includes people who definitely have Lyme disease, those with possible Lyme disease, and those who don't know what they have. One mother accompanied her daughter, who has an uncertain diagnosis, to a meeting. Afterward she wrote a letter saying it helped her understand what her daughter was going through to hear others discuss similar situations. I've talked with members of lupus, chronic fatigue, and MS support groups, and you can bet many of them can relate to what you're going through. Most sufferers of these diseases had symptoms for a long time before their own diagnosis and can identify well with your frustration.

When you're angry with God. When I was hospitalized for depression, one nurse urged me to pour out my anger at God. At the time I found it impossible to do because I could not feel any anger toward him, only a deep sense of confusion and fear. Others I have talked to said they felt much better after shouting at God for the "injustice" of what was happening to them. Some have experienced a degree of resolution and actually felt closer to God because of it.

My husband spouted his anger at God vehemently all the way to the hospital on one occasion in the midst of a particularly traumatic time in our struggle with my illness. He vowed that he was through praying and asking for God's help. However, within days after the episode he was soliciting prayers and attending a church service. If he had denied the anger he felt and stuffed it further inside, maybe it would have come out in much more destructive ways.

When you're angry with yourself. Anger with yourself for not holding up better might be the result of unrealistic expectations. It can take the form of guilt— blaming yourself for not being strong enough. Some days you will do better than others. You struggle along and try to hide your pain and fear, but it doesn't always work. No matter how strong you are, or how much religious faith you have, there are no guarantees you will always bear up under adversity. You will not always handle every situation well and say or do the right things. When you are ill you often respond more emotionally to incidents you normally would take calmly.

I thought I was a pretty strong person. I had certain expectations of the way I should respond to situations as a Christian. I later realized some of those expectations were unrealistic. My greatest agony for a long time was that I believed my credibility as a Christian had been destroyed by the suicide attempts and a severe depression that occurred during my illness. Yet so many others have said their faith has been strengthened through my sharing of the very things that for a time I believed had invalidated my faith. I am continually amazed at how beautifully God can work through the most painful experiences in life.

When you're angry with your friends. You will probably find that some of your friendships become more fragile when you have an ongoing illness. Everyone reacts differently. My friends found it very hard to understand why the doctors could find nothing wrong. They too held the misconception that if illnesses exist, they always show up on tests. Some of your friends will show concern at first, but fall away after awhile. Your anger might be due to a sense of rejection.

At the time when you feel you need them the most, some friends shy away. Handle your anger carefully. I lashed out at the one friend who indicated doubts about my illness, and I regretted it for years afterward. It was one instance where my impulsive expression of anger damaged a friendship. In all honesty I had to admit I might have had the same doubts had our situation been turned around. In my own pain I said some things that hurt her. If I had been able to discuss it more calmly, it might have spared us both a heartache.

When you're angry with your illness. Becoming furious with your illness is probably the most productive anger you can have. After all, it's the illness that has caused you so many problems in the first place. Such anger often precedes determination not to let it get the best of you. I found myself not just getting angry at my own pain, but at all the pain and suffering humanity endures. The illness was a constant reminder of the harsh reality that we can't always escape or control the bad things in this world. I often thought of my grandmother, who suffered severe heart damage from a bout with rheumatic fever. I recalled staying with her as a child and watching her struggle to make her way to the outhouse and back, gasping for breath and clutching her chest every step of the way. Every physical move she made took all the energy and stamina she could muster. I hated seeing her like that.

My great aunt was bedridden and suffered incredibly from a paralyzing disease for twenty years before she died. I had never met her but corresponded with her by mail. The reality of the depth of her pain hit home one day as I read through copies of her medical records. Not only was she paralyzed, her head was fixed permanently to one side, and her limbs were twisted in awkward positions. By the time I finished reading her case history, I was frightened and angry over the injustice of it all and scared to death that my illness could become that severe. It seemed so unfair that anyone would have to suffer so much for so long. I threw myself on the bed and cried. Then I determined not to let my own illness destroy my spirit.

Bargaining. When faced with a serious illness, people often go through a bargaining phase, promising to do better with their lives if only God will restore their health and give them another chance. Rather than bargaining for restored health, you might find that most of your bargaining centers around the issue of finding out what is wrong. "Dear God, if only I could know what is wrong, then I could start dealing with it. Maybe I could begin to find some purpose in this mess. If only I had a name for this illness, people would understand."

It is easy to believe that life would become much easier if you could validate your illness with a label. I thought I needed to have my illness confirmed before I could share my testimony or write about my experiences. I thought I needed some kind of prognosis before I could pursue any plans for the future. As time went by and test after test and doctor after doctor failed to provide answers, the realization set in that my bargaining was futile. Eventually I began sharing my testimony, writing my book, and finding ways to take college extension classes in spite of the obstacles the illness created.

Depression. This can be the most unwelcome of all aspects of the grieving process and the toughest to overcome. It often becomes an all-encompassing sense of despair, and keeping it under control can be an ongoing battle. When you become depressed over perceived losses— health, hope, dreams, and credibility— everything about your condition seems worse. Your will to survive plummets and you wonder whether it is worth fighting anymore. You no longer feel useful or worthwhile. You begin telling yourself your loved ones would be better off without you.

To make it, you need to be a fighter.

When negative thoughts and feelings cause your depression, you have a better chance of turning it around on your own. When changes in your body's metabolism resulting from the illness or drugs cause it, you may need professional care and possibly medication to help correct the imbalances.

Use the following suggestions to help yourself out of depression:

—Try not to become enveloped in self-pity.
It's hard not to feel sorry for yourself once in a while, but it won't help matters to harbor a "poor me" outlook permanently. Remind yourself that you are not the only one with problems. Those who are physically healthy have other ordeals to overcome. You have not been singled out to be afflicted. About one-third of the adult population in the United States suffers from some form of chronic illness.[2]

—Focus on the positive as much as possible.
Instead of telling yourself things will never get better,
remind yourself that time is a healer. You probably
have days when the symptoms are much more bear-
able than others. Tomorrow might be a better day.

—Focus on others around you.
Offer consolation or send a note of encouragement to
someone else who is struggling with another problem.

—Keep as physically active as possible.
Inactivity not only allows more time for you to dwell
on your suffering, it increases muscle weakness and
joint stiffness, which in turn lead to more pain. If
your strength is down, do just a little at a time.
Remember, too, the more active you are, the more
endorphins and other natural painkillers and antidepressants your brain will produce.

—Keep your mind occupied.
Scientific studies have shown that people who engage in mentally stimulating activities feel happier
and can measurably improve their physical health.[3]

When I was trying to overcome my depression, I
started picking unfamiliar words out of the dictionary and memorizing definitions in attempts to
distract myself from the fear and anxiety. It did help,
and I later appreciated the slight expansion of my
vocabulary.

I also read inspiring stories about others who had
overcome adversities, and after mentally repeating
"God hath not given us a spirit of fear, but of power
and of love and of a sound mind" (II Tim. 1:7) for
some time, it eventually became very real to me. I

overcame my fear and sense of helplessness and felt emotionally well.

— *Keep setting goals.*
Setting goals, even if they are small ones, will provide distraction from both the physical and mental pain. Goals as simple as resolving to get a letter written or inviting a friend over for coffee can provide a sense of purpose for the day.

— *Don't tell yourself you can't.*
Tell yourself you will try. You might surprise yourself at how much you can do. There were mornings when I woke up in so much pain I thought I could never make it through the day. But it never felt any better to lie in bed and dwell on it. More often than not, when I got up and busied myself with small tasks, I was able to accomplish more than I anticipated.

— *Don't project too far into the future.*
When everything seems overwhelming, learn to take on only one day or one small segment of a day (even five minutes). You only need to get through the next minute, then you can think about the next. Eventually each one will begin to get a little easier, and suddenly you will realize that time is moving at a good clip again. When I was in the middle of my depression, I promised myself I would never again complain if time started moving too fast. Now it is, and I am working to honor that promise.

When Depression Is More Than You Can Handle

No matter what causes your depression, if it becomes severe it is important that you seek help for it. If you are struggling with a sense of hopelessness and despair, feel as though you are losing control, or find yourself contemplating suicide, be sure to get professional help. When you are severely depressed it is impossible to believe things can get better, but they almost invariably do. With time and proper care people do get better.

Having been through episodes of both types of depression (endogenous and exogenous), I can vouch for the fact that in spite of your despair there is always hope. If you cannot believe that right now, let someone else believe it for you. The most significant thing that a counselor ever said to me when I was hospitalized for depression was, "Just because you feel this way now doesn't mean you always will." She was right! (See Chapter 8 for more discussion on depression.)

Fear and Anxiety

Fear and anxiety can either accompany depression or occur independently. When you don't know what is wrong with you, it is easy to fear the worst. Instead of being comforted that your tests show nothing, you worry that the doctors are missing something formidable and life-threatening.

At the onset of my illness, I had a real fear that I might die before they discovered what was wrong with me. I am sure my anxiety accentuated my symptoms. Over time I learned to relax more with them, reminding myself that, despite my worries, I was still here. I also came to grips with my mortality. I was going to die someday, regardless. In the meantime I resolved to live my life as fully as I could. If you can picture yourself in the worst possible scenario and face your fears head on, it might help you overcome those fears.

Acceptance

For many people acceptance and spiritual enlightenment are one and the same. Lil describes going through a time of feeling she was a tremendous burden on her family because of her illness. She questioned whether there was any purpose in her life: "I prayed and prayed about it and one day, all of a sudden, I got an awakening. I had heard about a younger person who was killed in an accident and I wondered why I was still here. Then I realized I'm here because the Lord chose me to be here. This is where I am and, believe it or not, I'm very happy." A rotating crew of volunteers who care for Lil during the day while her husband is at work attest to the fact that her happiness is contagious.

Many others have said that when they are able to reach a point of acceptance they become acutely aware of the good in life— their love is enhanced, they find joy in little things, and their peace overcomes fear and anxiety. Some even begin to look at their handicaps as a blessing because of what they learned through them. With renewed mental energy they find ways to improve the quality of their lives.

Adversity has a way of teaching all of us what is important and what is not. When you have dealt with the lack of credibility, the most important conclusion you will come to is that your belief in yourself is what counts most. When you have endured great pain, everything in life becomes relative, including what makes you feel worthwhile. Following a spinal tap I was completely debilitated by an excruciating headache. When the pain finally eased to the point I could sit upright long enough to tie my four-year-old son's shoes, I was ecstatic. I would never have believed that a minor task could bring me such an enormous sense of accomplishment. Accepting any chronic illness, whether diagnosed or not, involves accepting some degree of uncertainty. No one can ever know for sure how an illness will progress and what the long-term outcome will be. Experts can only offer probabilities and percentages, which are always subject to change and will always have exceptions.

When accepting an undiagnosed medical condition, you accept the uncertainty of the situation and the greater uncertainty of a condition with an unknown cause. You do not have percentages or statistics. In spite of this, you can determine to make the best of the situation and learn to take one day at a time. You can begin living more in the present than in the past or future. The more you can focus on other aspects of your life, the less importance the illness will have, and the more likely you are to find the "light and order" within yourself.

If you are struggling right now, I encourage you not to give up. When I was at the worst point of my illness and in the midst of a suicidal depression, if anyone had told me that life would someday be good again, I could not have believed it. But they would have been right.

Staying on Top

Once you reach a point of acceptance, it is important to work at keeping a positive outlook. It will be helpful if you take the following steps.

—Don't allow yourself to dwell on the things you can't do. Find things your energy level will permit you to do. I found that even though I had to pace myself and work slowly, I often was able to do most of my own housework. During those times when I could not, my children took care of the necessities, and I learned to let the other things go. More passive activities, such as reading, writing letters, and helping my children with homework, helped me feel worthwhile when I was too weak for any physical exertion.

—Keep setting goals and continue to work toward them. I had always hoped to return to school some day and get a college degree. For a while it seemed impossible. There were too many times I was unable to drive anywhere by myself. With the unpredictability of my illness, it was not likely that I would be well enough to attend without missing classes. And even if I was able to finish my degree, I had no idea what kind of career I would have the physical stamina for.

I finally signed up for one evening extension class offered in a nearby town. A friend was taking the class also, and I was able to ride with her. I continued to take one class at a time, finding people to ride with and studying at home when I was not well enough to attend. It felt good to be learning and focusing on aspects other than my physical discomfort. I realized it wasn't important or necessary to be guaranteed the ability to finish. The important thing was that I was trying, rather than resigning myself to thinking I could never do it.

—Take care of yourself. A good friend of mine has always taken time to do things for herself. Occasion-

ally, after a bit of self-pampering she would comment, "I'm worth it." At first I thought her rather egotistical. Yet, it later struck me that she is one of the most caring, thoughtful people I know and is quick to cheerfully offer assistance to anyone in need. Before my illness I had it in my head that it was not okay to think of myself, that others should always come first. I now believe we need to find a balance. Although I don't believe in selfishness, being too self-sacrificing often renders us less capable of caring for others and even resentful in the long run. When we care for ourselves, we can benefit ourselves and those around us.

When you are sick there are times when you need to be a little more self-centered. Say "no" to things you know will be too taxing and will sap your limited supply of strength. Save your energy for those things you feel are important. If you need to rest in the afternoon so you will be able to make dinner or attend an evening function, make sure you do it. You will be able to give more to others if you take care of your needs first.

— *Talk with others in similar situations.* Chances are, in talking with friends and relatives, you will hear of others who are in predicaments similar to yours. Through a friend I heard of another woman who was going through a similar ordeal. I asked for her address and dropped her a note. She was thrilled to hear from someone who could understand her situation, and we continued to correspond through the years. It really helps to unburden yourself occasionally to someone who knows where you are coming from. You may also check on support groups in your area. Many chronic illness sufferers will be familiar with your frustrations.

—*Laugh as much as possible.* I personally cherish
the ability to laugh, having lost it awhile during my
depression. It was the emotion that I missed expressing more than any other. I believed that, somehow, if I could regain my sense of humor, everything
else would be okay too.

Norman Cousins, who wrote the best-selling book,
Anatomy of an Illness, believes that laughter might
have been instrumental in his recovery from a very
painful, serious disease. He watched classic "Candid
Camera" films and old Marx Brothers movies from
his hospital bed and reports, "I made the joyous
discovery that ten minutes of genuine belly laughter
had an anesthetic effect and would give me at least
two hours of pain-free sleep."[4]

—*Learn to relax.* Learning to relax with your pain or
other symptoms will not relieve them completely, but
will make them much easier to deal with. You will
sleep better and you will cope with stress better.
When you are not relaxed, your muscles are tense,
which not only makes the symptoms worse, but uses
up energy. A variety of relaxation techniques have
been helpful to people dealing with pain and anxiety— meditation and prayer, biofeedback, progressive
relaxation, soothing tapes, warm baths, and mental
imagery. (See the appendix of this chapter for more
information on relaxation techniques.)

—*Remember to focus as much as possible on positive
things.* A verse in the Bible offers excellent advice:
"Fix your thoughts on what is true and good and
right— things that are pure and lovely, and dwell on
the fine good things in others. Think about all you
can praise God for and be glad about it." (Phil. 4:8)

—*Keep a journal.* Writing down your thoughts in a daily journal can relieve tension. According to Bernie Siegel, tests show that college students and executives who keep journals have more active immune systems and develop fewer colds and other illnesses during exam times and periods of work stress.[5]

—*Above all, remain hopeful.* After more than six years of illness, I did not believe I would ever have a name, let alone a successful treatment for my illness, but it happened! I know there are many who have suffered much longer than I did, and I wish all could be restored to health today. Yet none of us knows what lies around the corner. If today is a particularly bad day, tomorrow might bring something better.

I quoted the serenity prayer composed by Reinhold Niebuhr in my first book. I continue to find it calming and think it is worth quoting again:

> *God, grant me the serenity*
> *To accept the things I cannot change*
> *Courage to change the things I can*
> *And the wisdom to know the difference.*

Appendix to Chapter 10: Coping with Chronic Pain

Your illness will no doubt produce some degree of bodily tension whether it has been confirmed with a diagnosis or not. As we discussed in Chapter 8, tension and anxiety invariably make any physical condition worse by depleting precious energy resources, depriving you of sleep, and making you irritable. Learning to relax your mind and body can help you cope with your pain or other symptoms better. You probably will not be able to eliminate your symptoms entirely, but you will sleep better, minimize your pain, and find that you have more energy for productive activities if you can relax

Some people are able to learn to relax on their own. However, if you have been tense for a long time, you might not be aware that you are not relaxing. You can even forget what it feels like to be relaxed. Employing one or more relaxation techniques can help to break the cycle of tension and pain.

Psychological Techniques for Coping with Pain

People are sometimes resistant to trying psychological strategies for coping with pain because they assume the only kind of pain that will respond to these methods must be imagined pain. However, people with pain from known causes, even survivors of serious burns, have successfully employed mental pain-control techniques. In fact, it is psychogenic pain rather than physical pain that does not usually respond to any pain treatment at all because the patient needs the pain for some psychological reason.

Progressive muscle relaxation. This technique, developed by Dr. Edmund Jacobson, involves tightening muscles one at a time, then slowly allowing them to go limp and stay limp, noting the contrasting sensations. The process makes the participant more conscious of the feeling of relaxation and, with practice, allows the participant to relax at will.

By eliminating the muscle tightness that accompanies nervousness, anxiety, worry, irritability, and other undesirable states, it becomes possible to break the cycle of sleeplessness, increased pain, and even great tension that they tend to perpetuate. In an article on this subject, Leavitt Knight suggests starting with the large, easily controlled muscles, then moving on to the smaller ones. He states that for every minute you keep the larger muscles relaxed, more of the smaller ones will let go, even if you don't yet have the skill to relax the small ones voluntarily.[1]

At first it is best to practice progressive relaxation in a quiet place while lying on your back, but later you can do it even when you are up and about. You begin with your feet, curling your toes and tightening them as much as you can. Make yourself aware of the tension for several seconds, then allow the whole foot to relax completely, noting the difference in the way the muscles feel when they are relaxed. Continue alternately tightening and relaxing muscles in the legs, buttocks, abdomen, back, neck, jaw, hands, and arms. Once you have tensed and relaxed each set of muscles, lie still awhile, experiencing the calmness of being in a relaxed state. Once you have mastered the larger muscles you can work on the small ones, such as the muscles of the eye and mouth.

Many libraries and book stores have tapes available to help you learn this relaxation method. Knight stresses the importance of not giving up too soon, that it may take several months to learn to apply progressive relaxation effectively.

Controlled breathing techniques. Controlled breathing is a simple relaxation technique that enables you to slow your heart rate, lower your blood pressure, and relax tense muscles. Choose a quiet spot and relax all your muscles as much as you can. Then concentrate on breathing naturally through your nose. Keep your mouth closed, your jaw relaxed, and your teeth apart. As you breathe in and out, repeat the word "calm" silently. Each time your mind begins to wander, return your attention to your slow, relaxed breathing. In his book *Mastering Pain* Dr. Richard Sternbach recommends practicing controlled breathing for about twenty minutes twice a day at the same time and place each day.[2]

Biofeedback. Biofeedback teaches relaxation with the aid of special equipment. The equipment measures bodily processes you are not usually aware of, informs you instantly of what is occurring, and thus enables you to consciously modify the processes. The usual stress reaction to discomfort or pain involves an increase in adrenaline production. This leads to increased muscle tension, increased heart rate, and constricted blood vessels in the hands and feet. Biofeedback equipment will inform you of the degree of tension present in your body and reveals subtle increases and decreases in bodily tension, so you can learn to control it. If you are interested in trying biofeedback, you should talk with your physician. It seems to work best for those who have lost the ability to relax voluntarily and have not benefited from other methods.

Imagery. Various methods of guided imagery have helped some people to cope with their illnesses. By deliberately forming visual images in your mind of relaxed, peaceful places, or of your body in a well state, you can distract yourself from your physical discomfort. This is not much different from day-dreaming, except that it is more intentional. There is much current interest in the idea that focusing on positive images enhances the body's immune system, helping it to heal itself.

Some feel that guided imagery is simply hypnosis by another name, a form of putting oneself in a trance. However, Dr. Sternbach points out that guided imagery seems to help many who are not responsive to hypnosis.[3]

Other Methods of Pain Control

TENS (transcutaneous electrical nerve stimulation). A small, battery-powered device referred to as a TENS unit has proven effective in controlling pain, as well as other symptoms, in some people. The unit is not much bigger than a paging device and can be worn over a belt in a similar fashion. Electrodes taped to the body deliver electrical vibrations to the affected areas. These electrical impulses interrupt the injury signals the body is sending to the brain or spinal cord.

The long-term success rate of TENS varies, depending on the type of problem it is used for and the setting in which it is used. It is more effective for localized, rather than widespread, symptoms. When used for pain control alone, about 50 percent of pain patients receive significant relief from it, but the success rate declines to 30-35 percent after one year.[4] It seems to be more effective when patients use it in conjunction with more comprehensive pain-management programs.

TENS is sometimes also effective in treating symptoms other than pain. I used one to control chorea movement. I taped two electrodes to the side of my trunk that was involved and two below the nape of my neck because my head would turn from side to side. This worked quite well for several months, but eventually more muscles became involved and the movement seemed to extend beyond the unit's capabilities.

TENS involves very little risk. It is not addictive (although overuse can result in loss of effectiveness). Patients with cardiac pacemakers should not use it unless they are shielded against this type of electrical stimulation. Skin irritation from the tape can be a problem, but it will clear up when the tape is removed. TENS requires a doctor's prescription.

Medications. If carefully monitored, strong prescription analgesics are acceptable for short-term use to treat acute pain. However, long-term use of these drugs can lead to tolerance or addiction. With tolerance, changes occur within your body's cells, making it necessary for you to take higher and higher doses to attain the same amount of relief. If you become addicted, you will experience withdrawal symptoms when you discontinue the drug (usually the pain becomes much worse).

According to Dr. Sternbach, although most doctors prescribe strong analgesics "as needed" for pain, it is better to take a weak one to just take the edge off and to take them on a regular time schedule. People often wait until their pain becomes severe to take medication and then take the highest dose possible. However, Sternbach says that by taking the weakest effective analgesic on a continual basis, you will stay ahead of the pain and keep it from increasing. "There are now thousands of patients who were once taking the equivalent of eight to ten codeine tablets daily and still hurting alot, who are actually having less pain and taking only one or two aspirin (or aspirin substitute) three or four times daily— or taking nothing at all for pain."[5]

Sternbach goes on to explain that it is easier to deal with a constant level of pain than one that is always changing, especially when the pain is not severe. He stresses that the great majority of pain patients who have succeeded in overcoming their pain have given up on pain pills altogether.

Pain management programs. If you have not been successful in learning to manage your pain on your own, you might be interested in the organization and direction provided by one of the many pain clinics throughout the country. These clinics treat the pain problem by treating the whole person. They work on both the physical and emotional aspects of the problem— strengthening muscles, increasing activity, increasing relaxation, and encouraging healthy communication and behavior. Dr. Loran F. Pilling, founder of the Pilling Pain Clinic, describes the philosophy of his programs:

> *The most essential force in these programs that leads to healthy living is a trust relationship that is built up between the patients and the staff. A strong bond also develops among the patients*

who are all working toward healthy goals. Family involvement is essential to develop healthy communication again. A patient must spend weeks to months in a pain rehabilitation program to escape from the chronic pain syndrome, but this is a brief interlude compared to a lifetime of agonizing pain. God gave us pain to protect us from danger. It was never meant to be a disability.

If you and your doctor decide a pain-management program could benefit you, you might need to negotiate with your insurance company to determine how much of the cost it will agree to cover.

The American Chronic Pain Association in Sacramento, California, assists people in finding accredited pain-management clinics and provides information on chronic-pain support groups. The phone number is (916) 632-0922.

Additional suggestions. Avoid the use of stimulants, such as caffeine and nicotine, as these substances will increase muscle tension and blood pressure. Substances that contain caffeine include coffee, tea, chocolate, colas, and some nonprescription analgesics. If you feel better when you smoke and drink coffee, you are probably only calming withdrawal symptoms. In reality you are increasing your irritability, muscle tension, and restlessness.

CHAPTER 11

Relationships with Family and Friends

From its onset my illness threw my life and the lives of my family members into turmoil. Not just my body changed, every aspect of our lives changed. Our marriage changed. Family roles changed. Friendships changed. Our lifestyle changed.

Except for a few brief periods prior to the illness, I had run our household pretty much on my own. My husband worked long hours at his business. Even though I worked outside the home too, I took responsibility for household tasks, preparing meals, gardening, shopping, caring for and driving our four children to activities they were involved in. I was heavily involved in volunteer work. I had been the classic American supermom. Suddenly other people were taking over my roles, and it didn't seem right.

Many relatives and friends began stopping over on a regular basis, bringing meals and offering help with housework. Other people with whom we had previously spent a great deal of time stopped visiting or calling, and we missed them.

We all felt a deep sadness over the change from our familiar routine, sensing that somehow we could never recapture life as we had known it. We longed to have it back the way it was before. As desperately as we wanted to fix it, we couldn't. We all had to try to relearn how to effectively interact with each other and cope with our ever-changing situation.

Somehow my husband and I and our four children muddled our way through more than six years of unpredictable ups and downs. Even though I was never my former energetic self, after months of barely functioning there were several stretches when I appeared normal, but we never knew when things were going to get crazy again. On the surface we all started getting pretty matter-of-fact over the unpredictable illness that intruded on our lives, but inside everyone was hurting. We all had our own fears and longings.

It was not until after I was diagnosed and successfully treated for Lyme disease that our friends and relatives revealed concerns they had discussed among each other, but not shared with us. I was surprised how many said they thought I was dying and worried I would not see my children graduate.

Strangers who read our story frequently ask questions, such as "How is your family now?" and "What kind of scars did the ordeal leave?" When I tell them our family is still intact and there doesn't seem to be any residual damage to our psyches, some seem surprised. They tell me how fortunate we are. I know we are. Although the odds were against us, my husband and I believe we have a good marriage and positive relationships with our children, extended family members, and friends.

Other people have presented a number of different scenarios. Some say their marriages have fallen apart as a result of the inability of their partner to cope with their undiagnosed illness, and some have admitted being unable to forgive their spouse's lack of faith in them. One woman confided, "My husband would come home from work and find me lying on the couch in the afternoon, unable to get up and make dinner. After awhile he began to make sarcastic remarks about 'this illness of yours.' I couldn't deal with my symptoms *and* the fact that he didn't believe me anymore. We ended up getting a divorce."

To be doubted by the one person you are counting on and care about the most is tough. The resulting hurt often comes out as anger, defensiveness, and a tendency to misinterpret motives. The loss of trust is painful for both parties. A number of spouses of undiagnosed sufferers expressed their sense of helplessness and feelings of guilt. Susan said, "I vacillated between being angry and defensive toward the doctors for insisting there was nothing physically wrong with John and wondering if they could be right. Then I would feel guilty over my lack of faith in my own husband. It was tearing us both up emotionally."

Few stresses on relationships require a greater effort to understand and empathize, and a willingness to give and forgive than does a chronic undiagnosed illness. The overall divorce rate in the United States is 50 percent. That rises to 75 percent when either partner develops a chronic illness.[1] It is my guess that the strain on a marriage and family is even greater when the illness involves a lengthy prediagnosis stage.

Each person's situation is unique and requires different kinds of flexibility. The things that worked for us will not necessarily work for everyone. We had no guidelines to follow and neither will you. However, by reflecting on our personal experience and interviewing others I have gleaned a list of suggestions that might be of help to you:

When It Comes to Your Partner

— Understand that everyone has different ways of coping, and it might be very difficult for your spouse to express what he or she is feeling.

Early in my illness my husband often admitted feeling helpless, saying, "I just want you to be well again. I wish I knew what to do for you."

For Dan and Laura, the situation was different. When Laura became ill, Dan methodically took charge of tracking down the cause of her illness, but Dan found himself tuning out emotionally. It was two years before he was able to put into words that his deepest desire was to have her well again.

— Remember your spouse is grieving over many losses, too.

As Dan put it:

> Laura's illness required me to examine all the
> things that had been important to me up to that
> point. It threatened my financial plan, my social
> plan and my life. It was scary. I realized that
> everything we had worked to accomplish was
> going to fail. I had to go back and let go of those
> things one by one. It was like I was going on a
> journey and could bring only a limited number of
> items. I had to decide which ones were really
> important. Eventually I realized none of them
> were. I became content just being part of the
> fabric of life.

— *Don't expect your spouse to fulfill all of your needs.*

Laura discovered her illness brought out strengths
and weaknesses in each of them and that Dan could
not be her only source of support:

> Before the illness I had certain expectations of Dan.
> Eventually I realized that he couldn't fulfill all the
> roles I wanted him to. He wound up doing what he
> was best at—taking the problem-solving role by
> helping me find a diagnosis and treatment. I
> learned to rely on my kids and friends for emotional
> support when I needed it. The illness really brought
> out our differences, yet I realized that it didn't
> mean he didn't love me or that we couldn't handle
> the situation together.

Dan pointed out that he had a hard time figuring out
how to respond to Laura's ever-changing symptoms
and the moods that accompanied them. "She would
be worse for a while, then better, then worse again; I

couldn't figure out how I was supposed to treat her. Was she still my wife and partner or had she become a patient to care for?"

—As much as possible encourage your partner to continue participating in activities he or she enjoyed in the past, even if you can't always join in.

Jim and Betty had enjoyed doing things with their three sons until Jim's unexplained pain and fatigue often made it impossible for him to leave home. At first everyone's social life came to a standstill. Jim says, "When I was feeling lousy, Betty would hover around home and get weepy. I had to encourage her to get out and do things. I knew she was worried, but just because I was sick she didn't have to be miserable, too. When she did start getting out and doing things with the boys again, they came back home happy and started enjoying life again. It made me feel better, too."

—Focus on the things he or she is doing right.

There were times my husband came across as abrupt in regard to my illness and it hurt, but I would remind myself of all the times he had empathized, driven me to doctor appointments, and worked long hours to pay off medical bills. I knew I shouldn't be too hard on him. I tried to put myself in his position. If the tables had been turned, I'm sure my patience would have run out at times, too.

It is common with any ongoing illness for those who are close to you to be sympathetic at first, but as time goes by to become more aloof. Don't expect your partner always to anticipate your needs and be in tune to your suffering. He or she might need some distance to survive. Laura noted, "Sometimes Dan simply could not deal emotionally with the problems I was having and still function."

— *Understand that some doubts are inevitable.*

In talking to spouses of illness sufferers, most admit that at times during the prediagnosis stage they had doubts. So often doctors suggest or insist there is nothing physically wrong. When doctors seem so sure of themselves, it is confusing for everyone involved. In some instances the spouses had to consciously resolve to believe their ill partner. Dan remembers, "Early on it was very easy for me to doubt. However, I came to the conclusion I had trusted Laura for this long and I could continue to trust her concerning the illness. If I was going to deal with it, I had to trust in the process."

At one point my husband became suspicious about the reality of my symptoms. As much as I wanted him to believe in me, I knew he could not help feeling the way he did any more than I could help being sick. I confronted the situation by saying, "I can't change what is happening to me and I can't change what you think about it. I just need to know if you are going to stick with me or not." He affirmed that he was. It was helpful to establish that we were committed to stick it out together, in spite of the unanswered questions.

— *Be considerate of your spouse's feelings, but not to the point of neglecting your own needs.*

When my illness resulted in a movement disorder that caused uncontrollable jerking, my husband was reluctant to take me out in public. However, I knew I needed to get out in order to keep from sinking into depression, so I refused to stay home. In time, as most of our friends accepted my disorder and encouraged me to join them in outings, my husband became more comfortable with it too.

— Talk out your feelings with each other.

Very often anger at the illness will come out as anger at each other. On many occasions we were forced to leave social events early because of my symptoms, and sometimes my husband became surly. Talking about it reinforced that he was really upset at the illness rather than with me, which helped to prevent the anger from driving us further apart.

— Avoid making negative statements or apologizing for being sick.

Comments such as, "You would probably be better off without me," serve no useful purpose. If you are doing the best you can, there is no need to make apologies for what you cannot do.

— Reassure your spouse that he or she is helping you just by being there.

Feelings of helplessness can be overwhelming when someone you care about is sick. I frequently reminded my husband that his willingness to stick with me, his taking time to call and check on me from work, and his words of encouragement were helpful to me.

— Be willing to forgive.

I understand that some actions are intolerable and there are times marriages will not survive, but will-

ingness to forgive is probably one of the key ingredi-
ents in the survival of any relationship. It is unrealistic to expect people to always respond to you the
way you would like them to. At first my husband
was very attentive. He drove me to countless doctors' appointments and spent hours waiting for me
while I underwent medical tests. He occasionally
took it on himself to set up appointments.

As months and years went by and we continued to
spend time and money for nothing, his sense of
discouragement grew. When doctors told us repeatedly that nothing was showing up on tests, that
maybe I was neurotic, he became more and more
unsure what to believe. The illness was a huge
strain on our relationship and there were times when
I wondered whether we would make it. If I could
pinpoint one specific thing that was more responsible
for the survival of our marriage than any other, it
was probably that we never allowed ourselves to
consider divorce, even fleetingly. We were both
committed to the marriage "for better or for worse."

Responding to Your Children's Needs

How your children respond to your illness will depend a great deal on their ages, their individual
dispositions, and the severity of your symptoms.
Naturally, the more noticeably your condition affects
your ability to function, the greater impact it will
have on your children and the more role adjustments
they will need to make.

In my case, my symptoms initially put me out of
commission for several months. My children, who
were then four, eight, eleven, and thirteen, immediately found themselves shifting to unfamiliar roles.

They were all forced to become more responsible for their own care and each other's. My oldest son became more parent than sibling to the younger ones. When school started he made sure everyone was out of bed and ready to go before the bus arrived. He often acted as caretaker for me as well. On more than one occasion he had to pick me up off the floor and help me back to bed when I had collapsed. They all had to drop some activities they were involved in because they could no longer count on me to drive them around. My four-year-old learned to entertain himself during the day, make his own lunch, and clean up the kitchen after himself.

On the surface everyone seemed to deal with the changes quite well. However, underneath they all harbored unspoken fears about what was happening to me and its impact on their own lives. My youngest became more subdued and protective and often was reluctant to leave me. Teachers and school counselors later reported that the other children seemed more reflective and withdrawn during the roughest times.

Years down the road I was surprised to learn that my daughter had gone to the school librarian and her health teacher to ask for literature on illnesses she had heard mentioned. She seemed very matter-of-fact about my illness, but when I was finally diagnosed and treated, a lot of her pent up emotion came to the surface. Each year since, she remembers and reminds me of the exact date I started treatment.

It was very difficult to talk with our children about an illness that had no name, yet I realize now it would have helped to talk with them about their feelings.

The following are suggestions to help your children cope better with your illness.

— Open the door for them to ask questions and share their own fears.

Very often children harbor unexpressed fears. If you don't talk with them about your illness at all, they may take it as a morbid sign and imagine the worst. If you can encourage them to talk about their feelings, they at least will have the opportunity to express those fears and concerns. More than likely, their biggest worry is that you are going to die. I was surprised one day when my daughter blurted out, "Mom, do you have cancer?" I had been sick for about four years by then and there had been no mention of cancer at home. I had no idea how long she had been agonizing over that idea, but she seemed greatly relieved when I told her cancer was not the cause of my health problems.

It can be hard to offer reassurance about the future when you do not have a diagnosis. There will always be a number of possibilities that cannot be ruled out completely. It is important to be as open and honest about the situation as possible. Explain that some illnesses take a long time to diagnose. Admit that you don't know what is going to happen, and that even though doctors cannot fix everything, there are times when illnesses eventually get better on their own. Just because you are sick now does not mean you will stay sick forever.

— Encourage a sense of involvement.

Children often feel as helpless in the face of illness as adults do. Being able to do something to help might give them some sense of control. Laura tells of a time after a spinal tap in which a severe headache made it impossible for her to get out of bed or turn her head. Her teenage daughter took it upon herself to saw the legs off an old step ladder in order to place the television set at the right level for her mother to watch from bed without moving her head.

When my daughter was eight, she spent a lot of time making me get-well cards. By the time of my home IV treatment, she was thirteen and eager to help me by adjusting the rate of flow of medication into the IV tube. When your children offer help, let them know you appreciate their concern and that it does help you feel better.

— *Convey assurance that you are trying to find solutions.*

Dan and Laura say their three daughters were comforted in knowing they were not giving up. It was very important to them that their parents were continuing to search for solutions and for effective ways to deal with the problems the illness presented.

— *Explain your own reactions to your children.*

Let them know that sometimes illness makes you more irritable and depressed than normal, but that does not mean you don't care about them. We found that hugs became more important than ever.

— *Try to keep a sense of humor.*

There were times when my children and I all got the giggles over my strange gait and chorea movement. Even though they were still conscious of the serious side, being able to laugh about it relieved a lot of tension.

Things that Might Make You Feel Better as a Parent

—Don't dwell on what you no longer can do with and for your children.

Concentrate on what you still can do. I couldn't go out and play baseball or go biking, but I could enjoy hearing about their adventures, take rides in the car, and play board games.

—Realize that the increased responsibilities can be a positive experience for your child.

Out of necessity my children learned to do things I had always been in too much of a hurry to teach them— running the washing machine and cooking simple meals. When I returned home from one hospital stay, my daughter proudly announced she had learned to wash the floors. Those experiences were good for them and they learned to cooperate with each other better in the process.

—Remember that children are fairly resilient.

Children often understand and accept much more than we give them credit for. They appreciate honesty. When I was put on a drug that plunged me into a psychotic state, I attempted suicide twice. At first my husband was determined to keep what had happened from the children, but changed his mind. When he explained that the drug was responsible, they seemed to accept it very well. Later, when I decided to write about my experiences, they were all behind me. How much you tell your children will depend on their age and their ability to comprehend. If you are unsure, you may want to solicit help from a counselor.

Thoughts on Friendships

"I wish I could give you some of my strength," a friend said to me in the midst of my illness. I don't recall whether I answered out loud, but I do remember clearly that I was thinking at the time. If she only knew how much of her strength she had given me. She and so many other friends and family members gave so much of their time, their love, and their prayers. When I was ready to give up, they would not let me. They encouraged me, consoled me, and became angry for me. They believed in me when I didn't believe in myself. They not only gave me some of their strength, they literally became my strength and my faith. Because of what they did for me I have love and faith and strength to pass on to others.

Just as an illness causes changes in your immediate family, it will have an effect on everyone else who has been a part of your life, as well. If you were active in your community and had a busy social life before your illness, you will at first find a great many people are concerned about what's happening to you as they become aware of your health problems. They won't feel the impact of your illness as acutely as those who live with you every day, but nevertheless they will be affected in varying degrees.

I found that some people reacted with more intensity than I expected. I was blessed to have many caring relatives and friends who were generous in volunteering their time to chauffeur my kids, baby-sit for the younger ones while I was hospitalized, bring meals, send cards, and offer to help with laundry. I will be forever grateful, but at times even the kindness seemed like a mixed blessing. I worried about how I would ever repay them. I chastised myself, thinking I may not have been so willing to give up my time to help them if the tables had been turned. When the doctors started telling me my illness was a figment of my imagination, I questioned it myself and worried that I was putting my friends and family through a lot of trouble for nothing. I struggled with feelings of guilt.

There is no time in your life that the support of your close friends and extended family members is more important than when you are going through times of adversity. Keeping those relationships strong in the midst of undiagnosed illness will require patience and understanding on your part. Being able to react to and interact with friends and extended family in a constructive way during the prediagnosis stage is something you will have to learn through experience and perhaps trial and error.

Here are some points to keep in mind regarding your friendships.

— *Receiving help can also be a way of giving.*

Learning to graciously accept help when you need it and turn it down when you don't can be a real art. I found myself often feeling guilty for putting others out, yet worrying that if I turned down their offers I would hurt their feelings. Eventually I became comfortable accepting or asking for help when I needed it, realizing it made them feel good to do it. It also

became easier for me to thank people for their offers
and turn them down when I did not need help.

Lil Gibsen, a woman who lives in my town, is a
wonderful example of someone who has mastered the
art of accepting help. Stricken with multiple sclerosis, she is no longer able to even feed or dress herself
and relies on volunteers to care for her during the
day. She laughs and jokes with them and finds
delight in hearing about each of their lives. In return
for the time they give, her volunteer friends leave
with a sense that they, too, can rise above life's
tragedies with a joyful spirit.

*— When friends offer advice concerning medical care,
don't feel obligated to take it.*

Thank them for their concern, but don't feel you owe
it to them to try their particular remedies or resources. You need to do what feels comfortable for
you. I received a heap of conflicting advice on remedies and doctors. I appreciated the advice because
it assured me that my family and friends cared and
really wanted to help. I opted to explore some of the
suggestions but not others. I found that people were
usually not pushy and respected my choices.

— It is important to maintain two-way friendships.

Take an interest in your friends' activities, even if
you can't always participate. Remember to ask them
how they're doing and allow them to unload on you
once in a while. Listening might be one thing you
have more time for than you ever did before. Even
during the times I was unable to get out of bed when
people stopped by, I could provide a listening ear.
You can remain a sympathetic and affectionate
friend.

—Don't dominate conversations with the subject of your illness.

It is easy to become preoccupied with your illness while you are trying to figure out what's happening to your body. However, you are not going to resolve your illness by talking about it incessantly, nor will constant talking lend you credibility. You will only drive people away if you do that. Unless people indicate that they really want to know all the details, spare them. Chances are, the only people who will want to know everything about your illness are those who are going through similar situations and want to compare symptoms.

—Whether your illness has a name or not, no one is going to be able to completely understand what you are going through.

In her book *We Are Not Alone* Sefra Pitzele reveals that many of the same frustrations we encounter prior to the diagnosis of chronic illness may continue even after a diagnosis is established. So often those who are sick appear normal to those around them, making it easy for misunderstandings to occur. If some of your friends have a hard time understanding your illness, spend more time with those who make you feel good. One person told me she avoids a friend who seems to drag her down during her worst times, reserving the times when her symptoms temporarily wane to get together with that friend. You may need to seek out new friendships with others who are coping with undiagnosed problems. I learned of another woman in a situation similar to mine through a mutual friend. My own need for a sense of purpose prompted me to write her an encouraging note. She wrote back expressing her appreciation and we continued to correspond over the next several years. During my most discouraging moments, I knew I could count on her to lend a sympathetic ear, and vice versa.

CHAPTER 12

When Your Child Is the Victim

D uring the past few years I have received letters and calls from a number of parents whose children are suffering with undiagnosed medical problems. Their situation deserves to be addressed, yet when it came to writing this final chapter, a part of me hesitated. I rationalized that much of the information in this book applies to children as well as adults. The only difference is that, as the parent, you will need to be your child's advocate.

I was almost ready to scratch this portion entirely when a friend gave me the name of a couple who, when they learned about my project, expressed interest in talking with me. Brad and Lynn Schmidt are the parents of three boys, one of whom has an undiagnosed illness. After meeting them, it seemed right to include their story here.

At times Lynn sounded almost mechanical as she recounted the trauma of the past four years—years during which she and her husband, Brad, watched their son Matthew regress from a normal, bubbly, bright-eyed youngster who "laughed all the time" to a child with severe mental and physical limitations because of an illness that continues to defy explanation by medical experts. By now they have both relived the saga in their own minds a thousand times, trying to make sense of it all. And more than likely they have lost count of the number of times they have gone through every detail with doctors, hoping to provide a clue to the answer that would at least give them something to rest on and assure them they have done everything possible to help their son.

The first clue that something was going awry came when they turned to see Matthew slumped in his younger brother's lap in the back seat of the car on the way home from a Memorial Day picnic in 1987. From that day on they would never see six-year-old Matthew as they had known him.

During the next several days and weeks he began having grand mal seizures. Some lasted for hours. They occurred as often as ten times a day, and sometimes he stopped breathing. Between seizures Matthew experienced violent mood swings and hallucinations. At the children's hospital, test after test failed to explain the medical reason for his bizarre symptoms. The seizures were unrelenting and Matthew's health deteriorated. Brad and Lynn would have liked more opinions, but the doctor in charge informed them that Matthew was too sick to be transferred to another facility.

When Matthew was released from the hospital three months later he was still having uncontrollable seizures. During the times he was able to be up, he walked around in a stupor, not recognizing his parents or brothers. "He was like a little animal," Lynn recalls. His behavior became erratic. He threatened his mother with a knife and tried to jump out windows. Even with twenty-four-hour nursing care, it became necessary at times to tie him to his bed just so his caretakers could get some rest.

Brad and Lynn consulted other doctors and other clinics, tormented by the fact they still didn't know why all this was happening. "Before this happened, we were aware that doctors were limited, but it was still so difficult for us to comprehend that they couldn't come up with an answer for us," said Lynn.

At one point a roomful of doctors at the Mayo Clinic collectively determined that Matthew had Alper's disease, a rare, progressive, fatal neurological disease. His weight had plummeted so severely he looked as though he had been in a concentration camp. The Mayo physicians concluded Matthew would only survive a few more weeks and sent him home, asking the Schmidts to call them for an autopsy after his death.

Brad and Lynn discussed funeral plans with their minister and picked out a cemetery plot for Matthew. But he didn't die. After being on intravenous feedings for several days, Matthew started coming back, and it became obvious to his parents that he was not dying. "We had tried to convince the doctors he was simply starving because he wasn't able to eat. It was frustrating that they wouldn't listen to us. We felt like we were always trying to convince them of something and no one would believe us."

Three months after taking him home to die, Matthew's parents brought him back to the Mayo Clinic. The attending doctor was astonished when he saw Matthew had gained weight and strength. He admitted the earlier diagnosis of Alper's was an obvious mistake. The Schmidts hoped to receive advice on their next move but were disappointed. It seemed that once the doctors realized they had made a mistake they had nothing more to offer. "We really had the feeling they just wanted to get rid of us," Lynn recalled.

On their own Brad and Lynn began checking other alternatives, ending up at the University of Minnesota. They found a doctor who was willing to work with them on finding the best solution. That doctor eventually found ways to keep Matthew's seizures under better control with large doses of medication, but still was not able to provide answers as to the cause.

Of the myriad of tests done on Matthew, he tested positive only for Lyme disease and a past TB infection. However, all the doctors consulted insisted that neither disease was capable of causing the extreme symptoms he was having. They tried antibiotic therapy for a while, but there was no significant improvement in Matthew's condition. Brad and Lynn still wonder if the results would have been different if the antibiotics had been administered earlier.

Nearly four years after the onset of Matthew's illness, the Schmidts still have no answers. They only know that Matthew, now ten years old, functions on the level of a four-year-old, continues to have seizures, and needs constant care. Their lives are centered around caring for him and their other two sons, Tim, twelve, and David, eight. A lot of things have changed, including their perspective on life. Material things don't mean much to them now. Brad says things that used to seem stressful at work seem trivial. "There is just nothing that comes close to what we have already been through."

What is important to the Schmidts is their love for each other and for their children. Matthew is now able to attend special classes during the day, and Lynn has taken a job working with another handicapped child. Brad coaches Special Olympics and Matthew's brothers help. Lynn says the boys have become very sensitive to the needs of others and are the first to reach out to other children with problems. "The ordeal has brought out the caring side of all of us."

There are still times when it hurts so much to see Matthew struggle with the effects of seizures that Brad and Lynn wish he would have died. But Matthew has his sense of humor, offers hugs and kisses, and brings his parents joy. He doesn't remember anything before his illness. He only knows that he was sick "a big one."

The Schmidts have accepted their lot without bitterness toward anyone. Each of them reached a point of acceptance at different times, but both have a strong sense there is a reason for everything that has happened, and some day they will know why. They have a supportive and sympathetic minister and church.

If they could have done anything differently, they would have been more assertive with doctors from the beginning. They would have insisted on more opinions earlier. They realize they need to trust doctors to a certain extent, and they appreciate the care many have shown, but they now know how limited doctors are. They have talked with a few other parents in similar predicaments and wish a support group were available.

Following my interview with Brad and Lynn, I realized that perhaps the reason I had shied away from the issue of undiagnosed children was that I was unsure the conclusions I had drawn earlier would fit.

As difficult as my own struggle with undiagnosed illness was, the idea of watching one of my children go through a similar trauma was incomprehensible. If it meant sparing one of them, I would go through it all again. It was significant that, in the long run, everything Brad and Lynn learned from their experience paralleled my own conclusions. They affirmed that these things are true, whether it is yourself or your child who is suffering from an illness:

— *It is much harder when there is no name for it.*

The Schmidts say it would still bring them an enormous sense of relief to have a name for Matthew's illness.

— *It is possible to reach a point of acceptance even without a diagnosis.*

We will never be able to change or fix or have answers for everything. Although they say they will never give up on finding an answer, Brad and Lynn believe they can live with the situation. Finding an answer is no longer the dominant focus of their lives.

—It is possible to move beyond the anger and hurt and to forgive the mistakes of others.

Brad and Lynn became angry at times, but realized the importance of letting go of that anger and concentrating on the kindness of others.

—Good things can come out of any situation, no matter how bad.

Even though nothing else can touch the pain and suffering the Schmidt family endured, they have recognized many good things as a result of it: a closer family, a change of focus from material to spiritual values, and a greater love for each other and their fellow human beings.

—Love, hope and faith can provide a sense of joy and purpose in life in spite of the anguish.

Whether it involves yourself or your child, a life-changing illness will initiate an exploration of your spiritual values. Those who survive and find purpose almost invariably attribute their success to a belief in a caring God.

APPENDIX

Additional Resources

The most difficult aspect of dealing with an undiagnosed illness is the sense of isolation, the feeling that
no one else can really understand. So many of the
people who read my first book wrote to me, saying:
"Thank you, thank you, thank you for writing your
book. This is my story too." I have heard from
people who have been diagnosed with lupus, MS,
rheumatoid arthritis, Lyme disease, chronic fatigue
syndrome, and depression, as well as from those who
have been diagnosed with other conditions (rare and
common) and those whose symptoms remain a
mystery. Friends and relatives of victims have also
responded, saying they are able to empathize better
with a loved one after reading the book.

Just knowing that someone else in the world can
really understand you helps to lighten your load.
Several people in my area have expressed interest in
forming a support group for those with undiagnosed
illness, and I am currently in the process of organiz-
ing one. At this point I know of no other groups
specific to undiagnosed medical conditions. You may
want to consider starting a group in your area if you
have the time and energy. The number of support
groups people have organized to help others cope
with a variety of problems provides evidence that
they are filling a void. They are not only helpful to
victims but often take some of the burden from loved
ones. It is important to try to keep an upbeat atmosphere within the group and to focus on positive and
constructive issues rather than on negative ones.

Established Support Groups

If you do not wish to start your own support group you might want to check into established disease-specific support groups. It is not so important that the affliction be the same as yours; the most important thing is the group's attitude. It will be most helpful if you can find a group whose members can understand the difficult predicament you are in, promote healthy responses, and offer love and encouragement, rather than one whose members have a victim attitude and spend most of the time complaining. As you become more confident, you, in turn, might find reward in offering encouragement to others. The following is a list of some organizations that can help you locate support groups in your area whose members are likely to empathize with your predicament:

American Chronic Pain Association
    P.O. Box 850
    Rocklin, CA 95677

American Lupus Society, National Office
    23751 Madison Street
    Torrance, CA 90505

Arthritis Foundation-National Office
    1314 Spring Street, N.W.
    Atlanta, GA 30309

Chronic Fatigue Syndrome
    Association of Minnesota
    P.O. Box 24232
    St. Paul, MN 55124

The Lupus Foundation of America, Inc.,
National Office
P.O. Box 12897
St. Louis, MO 63141

The Midwestern Lyme Disease Association
3835 South 37th
Lincoln, NE 68506

National Multiple Sclerosis Society, National Office
208 East 42nd Street
New York, NY 10017

National Organization for Rare Disorders, Inc.
P.O. Box 8923
New Fairfield, CT 06812

National Self-Help Clearinghouse
Graduate School & University Center
of the City University of New York
33 West 42nd Street, Room 1227
New York, NY 10036

Pain Treatment Centers

The following organizations can assist you in finding
pain treatment centers closest to you, as well as
providing information on support groups:

American Chronic Pain Association
P.O. Box 850
Rocklin, CA 95677

National Chronic Pain Outreach Association, Inc.
8222 Wycliffe Court
Manassas, VA 22110

Information and Referrals

Many of the organizations mentioned in the above
sections also provide pamphlets with information
about specific diseases, and some have physician
lists. Most large hospitals also have information
lines staffed by nurses who are equipped to answer
medical questions, including where to turn for help
in dealing with various medical problems.

Chronic and Undiagnosed Illness Counseling Services

In Minnesota only, Joyce Abel, a certified adult nurse
practitioner and licensed independent clinical social
worker, has a private practice offering individual and
group therapy for people with ongoing and undiagnosed illness. She also acts as a consultant to
people in the process of putting a medical team
together and co-leads a group along with a hospital
chaplain for those who are interested in exploring the
spiritual issues presented by illness. For more
information or appointments, call (612) 925-9276.

Miscellaneous Addresses

National Association of the
Physically Handicapped
2810 Terrace Road, SE
Washington, DC 20020

National Rehabilitation Information Center
The Catholic University of America
4407 Eighth Street, NE
Washington, DC 20017

Vocational Guidance and Rehabilitation Services
2289 East 55th Street
Cleveland, OH 44103

Information on Patients' Rights

Inquiries or complaints regarding medical treatment or about the patients' bill of rights may be directed to your state board of medical examiners or the office of health facility complaints.

Suggested Reading

Fisher, Gregg Charles. *Chronic Fatigue Syndrome: A Victim's Guide to Understanding, Treating and Coping with This Debilitating Illness.* New York: Warner Books, 1989.

Hanner, Linda. *Lyme Disease: My Search for a Diagnosis.* Maple Plain, MN: Kashan Publishing, 1989.

Hilfiker, David. *Healing the Wounds: A Physician Looks at His Work.* New York: Pantheon Books, 1985.

Huttmann, Barbara, R.N. *The Patient's Advocate: The Complete Handbook of Patient's Rights.* New York: Penguin Books, 1981.

Katz, Jay, M.D. *The Silent World of Doctor and Patient.* New York: The Free Press, 1984.

Pitzele, Sefra Kobrin. *One More Day: Daily Meditations for the Chronically Ill.* Minneapolis, Minnesota: Hazelden, 1988.

Pitzele, Sefra Kobrin. *We Are Not Alone: Learning to Live with Chronic Illness.* New York: Workman, 1985.

Weil, Andrew, M.D. *Health and Healing: Understanding Conventional and Alternative Medicine.* Boston: Houghton Mifflin, 1983.

Radzuina, Eileen. *Lupus: My Search for a Diagnosis.* Claremont, CA: Hunter House, 1989.

Register, Cheri. *Living with Chronic Illness: Days of Patience and Passion.* New York: Free Press, 1987.

Siegel, Bernie S., M.D. *Peace, Love & Healing.* New York: Harper & Row, 1989.

Sternbach, Dr. Richard A. *Mastering Pain: A Twelve-Step Program for Coping with Chronic Pain.* New York: Ballantine Books, 1987.

Thornhill, Annette. *Ask Your Doctor, Ask Yourself.* Gloucester, MA: Para Research, 1986.

References

CHAPTER 1

1. Robertson, Ian. *Sociology*, 3rd ed. (New York: Worth Publishers, Inc., 1987), 440.

CHAPTER 2

1. Harvey, A.M., Bordley, J, III, Barondess, J.A. *Differential Diagnosis*, 3rd ed., (Philadelphia: W.B. Saunders Co, 1979), 1.

2. Inlander, C.B., Lenn, L.S., Werner, E. *Medicine on Trial* (New York: Prentice Hall Press, 1988), 42.

3. Bradwell, A.R., Carmalt, M.H.B., Whitehead, T.P. Explaining the Unexpected Abnormal Results of Biochemical Profile Investigations. *Lancet*, Nov. 2, 1974, 1071.

4. Hutton, J.J., Kohler, P.O., O'Rourke, R.A., et al. *Internal Medicine*, 3rd ed. Boston: Little, Brown & Co., 1990), 1744-5.

5. Ibid., 1969,

6. Ibid., 1533.

7. Ibid.

8. Smith, B.E., Dyck, P.J. Peripheral Neuropathy in the Eosinophilia-Myalgia Syndrome Associated with L-Tryptophan Ingestion. *Neurology*, July 1990, 1038.

1. Siegel, Bernie S., M.D. *Peace, Love & Healing* (New York: Harper & Row, Publishers, 1989), 20.

2. Katz, Jay, M.D. *The Silent World of Doctor and Patient* (New York: The Free Press, 1984), 191-192.

3. Weil, Andrew, M.D. *Health and Healing: Understanding Conventional and Alternative Medicine,* (Boston: Houghton Mifflin Co., 1983), 210.

4. Siegel, *Peace, Love & Healing,* 253.

5. Weil, *Health and Healing,* 149.

6. Sternbach, Dr. Richard A. *Mastering Pain: A Twelve-Step Program for Coping with Chronic Pain,* (New York: Ballantine Books, 1987), 51.

7. Ibid., 51.

8. Weil, *Health and Healing,* 150.

9. Thornhill, Annette. *Ask Your Doctor, Ask Yourself,* (Gloucester, MA: Para Research, 1986), 102.

10. Ibid.

11. Weil, *Health and Healing,* 132.

12. Gibney, Michael J. *Nutrition, Diet & Health,* (Cambridge, MA: Cambridge University Press, 1986), 75.

13. Ibid., 82.

14. Ibid., 78-79.

15. Ibid., 79.

16. Ibid., 82.

17. Jones, Bob E. *The Difference a Doctor of Osteopathy Makes* (Oklahoma City, OK: Times-Journal Publishing, 1978).

18. Thornhill, *Ask Your Doctor, Ask Yourself,* 109.

19. Weil, *Health and Healing,* 127-128.

20. Panos, Maesimund B. *Homeopathic Medicine at Home,* (Los Angeles: Jo P. Tarcher, 1981).

21. Weil, *Health and Healing,* 33, 34.

22. Ibid., 32.

23. Ibid., 182.

CHAPTER 4

1. Radziunas, Eileen. *Lupus: My Search for a Diagnosis,* (Claremont, CA: Hunter House, 1989), xii-xiii.

CHAPTER 5

1. Radziunas, Eileen. *Lupus: My Search for a Diagnosis,* (Claremont, CA: Hunter House, 1989), 26.

2. Gillespie, Larrian, M.D., *You Don't Have to Live with Cystitis! How to Avoid It, What to Do About It,* (New York: Avon Books, 1988), 114.

3. Ibid., 114.

1. Hilfiker, David. *Healing the Wounds: A Physician Looks at His Work* (New York: Pantheon Books, 1985), 197.

2. Ibid., 50.

3. Ibid., 77.

4. Ibid.

5. Ibid., 85.

6. Siegel, Bernie S., M.D., *Peace, Love & Healing* (New York: Harper & Row, 1989), 130, 132.

7. Hilfiker, *Healing the Wounds*, 70.

8. Feinstein, Alvan.*Clinical Judgment* (Baltimore: Williams & Williams Co., 1967), 23-24.

9. Siegel, *Peace, Love & Healing*, 227.

10. Katz, Jay, M.D., *The Silent World of Doctor and Patient*, (New York: The Free Press, 1984), 102.

11. Huttmann, Barbara, R.N., *The Patient's Advocate: The Complete Handbook of Patient's Rights* (New York: Penguin Books, 1981), 185.

12. Siegel, *Peace, Love & Healing*, 227.

CHAPTER 7

1. Huttmann, Barbara, R.N. *The Patient's Advocate: The Complete Handbook of Patient's Rights* (New York: Penguin, 1981), 185.

2. Annas, George J. *Judging Medicine* (Clifton, NJ: Humana Press, 1988), 10.

3. Huttmann, *The Patient's Advocate*, 277-278.

4. Ibid., 278.

5. Thornhill, Annette. *Ask Your Doctor, Ask Yourself* (Gloucester, MA: Para Research, 1986), 48.

6. Ibid., 41.

7. Dowie, Mark, et al., "The Illusion of Safety," *Mother Jones Magazine*, 7 (June 1982): 47.

8. Illich, Ivan. *Medical Nemesis: The Expropriation of Health* (New York: Pantheon Books, 1982), 70-71.

9. Cousins, Norman. *Anatomy of an Illness as Perceived by the Patient: Reflections on Healing and Regeneration* (New York: Bantam Books, 1981), 44.

10. Weil, Andrew, M.D., *Health and Healing: Understanding Conventional and Alternative Medicine* (Boston: Houghton Mifflin, 1983), 16.

11. Ibid., 110.

12. Thornhill, *Ask Your Doctor, Ask Yourself*, 83.

CHAPTER 8

1. Barsky, Arthur J. *Worried Sick: Our Troubled Quest for Wellness* (Boston: Little, Brown, 1988), 22.

2. Beecher, H.K. "Relationship of Significance of Wound to Pain Experience," *Journal of the American Medical Association* 161 (1956): 1609-1613.

3. Holmes, Thomas H., M.D., and Rahe, Richard H., M.D., "Holmes-Rahe Social Readjustment Rating Scale." *Journal of Psychosomatic Research,* 11 (1967): 214-218.

CHAPTER 9

1. Radziunas, Eileen. *Lupus: My Search for a Diagnosis* (Claremont, CA: Hunter House, 1989), xii.

CHAPTER 10

1. Miller, William A. *Why Do Christians Break Down?* (Minneapolis, MN: Augsburg Publishing House, 1973), 45.

2. Pitzele, Sefra Kobrin . *We Are Not Alone: Learning to Live with Chronic Illness* (New York: Workman Publishing, 1985) 15-16.

3. Katz, Nancy. "Nimble Minds Make Nimble Joints." *Arthritis Today,* (Jan-Feb. 1991): 44.

4. Cousins, Norman. *Anatomy of an Illness* (New York: Bantam Books, 1981) 11, 39.

5. Siegel, Bernie S., M.D., *Peace, Love & Healing* (New York: Harper & Row, 1989), 224.

6. Knight, Leavitt A., Jr. "How to Relax Without Pills." *The American Legion Magazine* (Oct. 1970): 14.

7. Sternbach, Dr. Richard A. *Mastering Pain: A Twelve-Step Program for Coping with Chronic Pain* (New York: Ballantine Books, 1987), 101-102.

8. Ibid., 99.

9. Ibid., 146.

10. Ibid., 139-140.

CHAPTER 11

1. Pitzele, Sefra Kobrin. *We Are Not Alone: Learning to Live with Chronic Illness* (New York: Workman Publishing, 1985), 15, 16.

Bibliography

Annas, George J. *Judging Medicine.* Clifton, NJ: Humana Press, 1988.

Barsky, Arthur J. *Worried Sick: Our Troubled Quest for Wellness.* Boston: Little, Brown, 1988.

Beecher, H.K. "Relationship of Significance of Wound to Pain Experience," *Journal of the American Medical Association* 161 (1956):1609-1613.

Boston Women's Health Collective. *Our Bodies, Ourselves.* New York: Simon & Schuster, 1989.

Cheraskin, M.D., D.M.D. *The Vitamin Controversy: Questions & Answers.* Witchita, KS: Bio-Communications Press, 1988.

Cousins, Norman. *Anatomy of an Illness as Perceived by the Patient: Reflections on Healing and Regeneration.* New York: Bantam Books, 1981.

Davis, Joel. *Endorphins: New Waves in Chemistry.* Garden City, NY: The Dial Press, 1984.

Dowie, Mark. "The Illusion of Safety," *Mother Jones Magazine* 7 (June 1982).

Feinstein, Alvan. *Clinical Judgment.* Baltimore: Williams & Williams Co., 1967.

Gibney, Michael J. *Nutrition, Diet & Health.* Cambridge, MA: Cambridge University Press, 1986.

Gillespie, Larrian, M.D. *You Don't Have to Live with Cystitis! How to Avoid It, What to Do About It.* New York: Avon Books, 1988.

Harvey, A.M., Bordley, J, III, Barondess, J.A. *Differential Diagnosis,* 3rd ed., Philadelphia: W.B. Saunders Co, 1979.

Hilfiker, David. *Healing the Wounds: A Physician Looks at His Work.* New York: Pantheon Books, 1985.

Holmes, Thomas H., M.D. "Holmes-Rahe Social Readjustment Rating Scale," *Journal of Psychosomatic Research* 11 (1967): 214-218.

Huttmann, Barbara, R.N. *The Patient's Advocate: The Complete Handbook of Patient's Rights.* New York: Penguin, 1981.

Illich, Ivan. *Medical Nemesis.* New York: Pantheon Books.

Inlander, C.B., Lenn, L.S., Werner, E. *Medicine on Trial* New York: Prentice Hall Press, 1988.

Jones, Bob. *The Difference a Doctor of Osteopathy Makes.* Oklahoma City, OK: Times-Journal Publishing, 1978.

Katz, Jay, M.D. *The Silent World of Doctor and Patient.* New York: The Free Press, 1984.

Katz, Nancy. "Nimble Minds Make Nimble Joints," *Arthritis Today* (Jan-Feb 1991): 44.

Knight, Leavitt A. "How to Relax Without Pills," *The American Legion Magazine* (Oct. 1970): 14.

Knowles, John H., Ed. *Doing Better and Feeling Worse: Health in the United States.* New York: W.W. Norton, 1977.

Long, Patricia. *The Nutritional Ages of Women: A Lifetime Guide to Eating Right for Health, Beauty, and Well-Being.* New York: MacMillan, 1986.

Miller, William A. *Why Do Christians Break Down?* Minneapolis, MN: Augsburg Publishing, 1973.

Panos, Maesimund B. *Homeopathic Medicine at Home.* Los Angeles: J.P. Tarcher, 1981.

Pinckney, Cathey and Edward R. *Do-It-Yourself Medical Testing: More than 160 Tests You Can Do at Home.* New York: Facts-on-File Publications, 1983.

— .*The Encyclopedia of Medical Tests.* New York: Facts-on-File Publications, 1983.

— .*The Patient's Guide to Medical Tests.* New York: Facts-on-File Publications, 1982.
Pitzele, Sefra Kobrin. *We Are Not Alone: Learning to Live With Chronic Illness.* New York: Workman, 1985.

Radziunas, Eileen. *Lupus: My Search for a Diagnosis.* Claremont, CA: Hunter House, 1989.

Robertson, Ian. *Sociology,* 3rd ed. New York: Worth Publishers, 1987.

Siegel, Bernie S., M.D. *Peace, Love & Healing.* New York: Harper & Row, 1989.

Sternbach, Dr. Richard A. *Mastering Pain: A Twelve-Step Program for Coping with Chronic Pain.* New York: Ballantine Books, 1987.

Thornhill, Annette. *Ask Your Doctor, Ask Yourself.* Gloucester, MA: Para Research, 1986.

Weil, Andrew, M.D. *Health and Healing: Understanding Conventional and Alternative Medicine.* Boston: Houghton-Mifflin, 1983.

INDEX

Acceptance, 179-180
Acquired immunodeficiency syndrome, 29
Acupuncture, 39-40
AIDS, 29
Allergist, 58
Alternative therapies, 36-52
American Chronic Pain Association, 191
Amplifiers of symptoms, 130-132
Analgesics, 35, 189-190
Anger, 166-174
      constructive, 168-170, 173-174
      with doctors, 167-170
      with friends, 172-173
      with God, 171-172
      with the illness, 173-174
      with spouse and family, 170-171, 195-196
      with yourself, 172
Angiography, 106
Annas, George J., *Judging Medicine*, 97
Anxiety, 17, 162, 178-179
Ask Your Doctor, Ask Yourself (Thornhill), 123

Bargaining, 174-175
Believing in yourself, 157-159
Biofeedback, 187
Blaming the victim, 7
Brainstem Auditory Evoked Response (BAER), 109
Breathing, 187

Cardiologist, 59
CAT Scan, 106
Children with undiagnosed illness, 211-217
Chiropractic, 41-42

Doing nothing, 32-33
Drugs. See Medication

Electrocardiography (ECG), 108
Electroencephalography (EEG), 108
Electromyography (EMG), 108
Emotions, 125-126, 162, 163, 164-179
Encyclopedia of Medical Tests (Pinckney), 111
Endocrinologist, 59
Evoked Responses, 108-109

Fear, 162, 178-179
Feelings. See Emotions
Feinstein, Alvan, *Clinical Judgment*, 88-89

Gastroenterologist, 59
Geriatrician, 58
Grieving process, 162-163
Gynecologist, 58

Healing the Wounds (Hilfiker), 80, 82, 87-88, 92
Hematologist, 59
Hilfiker, David, *Healing the Wounds*, 80, 82,
    87-88, 92
History, medical, 16-17
Holistic medicine, 49-50
Homeopathy, 47-48
Hospital Experience, The (Nierenberg), 111
Huttmann, Barbara, *The Patient's Advocate*, 92-93,
    98
Hypochondriasis, 142

Imagery, 188
Infectious disease specialist, 59
Internist, 59

Judging Medicine, (Annas), 97

DCI Publishing Books of Related Interest

❑ **The Physician Within** by Catherine Feste. Here internationally renowned health motivation specialist, Cathy Feste, focuses on motivating
those with a health challenge, and anyone else, to stay on their regimen and
follow healthy behavior.

004019, ISBN 0-937721-19-0, $8.95

❑ **Whole Parent/Whole Child: A Parents' Guide to Raising a Child
with a Chronic Illness** by Patricia Moynihan, RN, PNP, MPH, and Broatch
Haig, RD, CDE. Everything parents of children with chronic health conditions need to know is here. With authority, insight, and compassion, this
book shows you how to be the kind of parent you want to be and how to
help your child lead the fullest life possible.

004051, ISBN 0-937721-53-0, $9.95

❑ **I Can Cope: Staying Healthy with Cancer** by Judi Johnson, RN, PhD,
and Linda Klein. This book is a clear, comprehensive resource for anyone
whose life has been touched by cancer. And it's by Judi Johnson, co-
founder of the American Cancer Society's internationally acclaimed "I Can
Cope" program, which helps over 40,000 people a year.

004026, ISBN 0937721-28-X $8.95

❑ **Making the Most of Medicare: A Personal Guide Through the
Medicare Maze** by Arthur R. Pell, PhD. Finally a book that actually helps
overcome the government red tape associated with Medicare. It shows what
can and cannot be expected from Medicare and provides easily understood
explanations of Medicare policies—plus tips on how to use them for opti-
mum advantage.

004071 ISBN 0-937721-66-2, $11.95

❑ **Retirement: New Beginnings, New Challenges, New Successes** by
Leo Hauser and Vincent Miller. From two internationally renowned motiva-
tional speakers, trainers, and retirees comes a book that will help you
achieve new goals in retirement. It's a plan of action that charts a course to
successful, rewarding, and active retirement.

004059, ISBN 0-937721-59-X, $5.95

❑ **Fast Food Facts** by Marion Franz, RD, MS. This revised and up-to-date
best-seller shows how to make smart nutritional choices at fast food restaurants—and tells what to avoid. Includes complete nutritional information on
over 1,000 menu offerings from the 32 largest fast food chains.

Standard size edition   004068, ISBN 0-937721-67-0, $6.95
Pocket edition   004073, ISBN 0-937721-69-7, $4.95

❑ **All-American Low-Fat Meals in Minutes** by M.J. Smith, RD, LD, MA. Filled with tantalizing recipes and invaluable tips, this cookbook makes great tasting low-fat foods a snap for holidays, special occasions, or every day. Most recipes take only minutes to prepare.

004079, ISBN 0-937721-73-5, $12.95

❑ **Exchanges for All Occasions** by Marion Franz, RD, MS. Includes exchanges and meal planning suggestions for just about any occasion, sample meal plans, special tips for people with diabetes, and more.

004003, ISBN 0-937721-22-0, $8.95

❑ **Fight Fat & Win** by Elaine Moquette-Magee, RD, MPH. This break-through book explains how to easily incorporate low-fat dietary guidelines into every modern eating experience, from fast food and common restaurants to quick meals at home, simply by making smarter choices.

004070, ISBN 0-937721-65-4, $9.95

❑ **The Expresslane Diet** by Audrey Fran Blumenfeld, RD. This 21-day weight-management plan meets U.S. recommended daily allowances using brand name convenience and frozen foods and even some fast foods. With this nutritious diet you'll lose weight quickly—up to seven pounds a week.

004055, ISBN 0-937721-61-1, $7.95

_____

Buy them at your local bookstore or use this convenient coupon for ordering.

DCI Publishing
P.O. Box 47945
Minneapolis, MN 55447-9727

Please send me the books I have checked above. I am enclosing $_____. (Please add $2.50 to this order to cover postage and handling. Minnesota residents add 6% sales tax.) Send check or money order, no cash or C.O.D.'s. Prices are subject to change without notice.

Name _____

Address _____

City _____ State _____ Zip Code_____

Allow 4 to 6 weeks for delivery.
Quantity discounts available upon request.

Or order by phone: 1-800-848-2793,
1-800-444-5951 (non-metro area of Minnesota)
612-541-0239 (Minneapolis/St. Paul metro area).

Please have your credit card number ready.